Medical Mycology

A Self-Instructional Text
2nd Edition

Martha E. Kern, MD, DA, MT(ASCP), CLS(NCA)
Vice Chairman, Internal Medicine
Suburban Hospital
Bethesda, Maryland

Kathleen S. Blevins, PhD, MT(ASCP), CLS(NCA)
Assistant Professor of Research
The University of Oklahoma Health Sciences Center
College of Public Health
Center for American Indian Health Research
Oklahoma City, Oklahoma

F. A. DAVIS COMPANY • Philadelphia

F. A. Davis Company
1915 Arch Street
Philadelphia, PA 19103

Printed in the United States of America

Last digit indicates print number: 10

Publisher: Jean-François Vilain
Developmental Editor: Crystal Spraggins
Production Editor: Jessica Howie Martin
Cover Designer: Louis J. Forgione

As new scientific information becomes available through basic and clinical research, recommended treatments and drug therapies undergo changes. The authors and publisher have done everything possible to make this book accurate, up to date, and in accord with accepted standards at the time of publication. The authors, editors, and publisher are not responsible for errors or omissions or for consequences from application of the book, and make no warranty, expressed or implied, in regard to the contents of the book. Any practice described in this book should be applied by the reader in accordance with professional standards of care used in regard to the unique circumstances that may apply in each situation. The reader is advised always to check product information (package inserts) for changes and new information regarding dose and contraindications before administering any drug. Caution is especially urged when using new or infrequently ordered drugs.

Library of Congress Cataloging-in-Publication Data

Kern, Martha E.
    Medical mycology : a self-instructional text / Martha E. Kern, Kathleen
S. Blevins.—2nd ed.
      p. cm
    Includes bibliographical references and index.
    ISBN 10: 0-8036-0036-4 (pbk.) ISBN 13: 978-0-8036-0036-2
    1. Medical mycology—Programmed instruction. I. Blevins,
Kathleen S. II. Title.
    [DNLM: 1. Fungi—programmed instruction. 2. Mycoses—programmed
instruction. 3. Microbiological Techniques—programmed instruction.
QW 18.2 K39m 1997]
QR245.K47 1997
616.9'69—dc21
DNLM/DLC
for Library of Congress   96-46605
                                 CIP

Preface to the Second Edition

Since the first edition of this text, medical science has made breakthroughs in technology, and complex procedures—including organ and bone marrow transplants, cardiac balloon angioplasties, and cancer chemotherapy—have become commonplace. As a result, patients are not only living longer but living in an immunocompromised state and demonstrating all of the attendant infectious sequelae. In addition, new immunologically debilitating diseases such as AIDS have surfaced to challenge our therapies. It is ever more important to rapidly identify previously uncommon diseases and to treat them appropriately.

This edition features the new technology as it relates to rapid identification of fungal organisms and antifungal therapy. Manual identification protocols in the first edition have been replaced with discussions of commercial and automated identification systems, especially for blood culture and yeast speciation. The section on seromycology now emphasizes kits for *Candida* and *Cryptococcus* antigen testing from clinical specimens. Advantages and pitfalls of exoantigen testing and DNA probes are elucidated. All fungal names have been updated, and newly recognized opportunistic pathogens are included, such as *Penicillium marneffei, Apophysomyces elegans, Saksenaea vasiformis,* and *Scedosporium prolificans.* Diseases are discussed with particular organisms or groups of organisms instead of in separate "Supplemental Rationale" sections. Updated disease descriptions include one of AIDS patients, who sometimes do not exhibit classic disease manifestations. There is a new section on antifungal antibiotics, with a discussion of antibiotic resistance.

The text includes new photographs, and charts are incorporated throughout the modules rather than at the end of each module. The self-tutorial format is maintained, with updated study questions. The content outlines make it easy to follow through the modules, while objectives and follow-up activities complete the text. Bibliographies have been updated.

We believe this edition responds to today's needs. It includes numerous helpful suggestions from educators and technologists, and we expect that this book will be an aid to both.

Martha E. Kern
Kathleen S. Blevins

Preface to the First Edition

Fungi have always been a plague to man. Of the 200,000 or more species that exist, approximately 100 of them consistently produce human mycoses. Most pathogenic fungi elicit chronic infections of the superficial, cutaneous, and subcutaneous tissues, causing unsightly but not lethal diseases. In the past, systemic infections were infrequent and usually confined to patients with naturally deficient immune mechanisms or debilitating disease. Recently, however, with increased use of immunosuppressive drugs, antibiotics, and chemotherapy, disseminated life-threatening mycoses are more frequently observed. In addition to classic systemic pathogens, the causative agents are often opportunistic fungal contaminants that previously held no significant disease association.

A competent laboratory mycologist must be aware of the changing etiologic role of fungi. Without proper specimen collection, processing, and culture methods, potential pathogens may be completely missed, with fatal consequences to the patient.

Just as important, the technologist must be able to correctly identify causative organisms within a time frame useful to the clinician and the patient. Since many fungi require a long growth period, a thorough, accurate examination of the specimen direct mount is imperative. It provides a rapid presumptive diagnosis upon which the physician can act. For final mycologic identification, relatively few physiologic tests are available. Differentiation between morphologically similar fungi basically depends on the technologist's experience and judgment. To someone just entering the field, the melange of subleties in appearance may prove very frustrating.

Many volumes containing fungal descriptions and procedures have been written. Unfortunately, most of them are too detailed and technically oriented to be appropriate for the beginning mycology student. In addition, laboratory technology and microbiology training curricula are so condensed that little time is available for mycologic instruction. The purpose of this book is to provide a basic and practical course in laboratory mycology that can be used for self-teaching or as an adjunct for instructors. The volume also fits the needs of clinical mycology laboratories. Each module contains text with drawings, photographs, and charts. Incorporated into the text are a series of self-study examinations that encourage the reader to actively participate in the learning process. Each unit also contains prerequisites, behavioral objectives, a content outline, follow-up activities, and selected references. All modules except Module 4 contain a Supplemental Rationale section which includes material that is valuable to know but not absolutely necessary for day-to-day laboratory work. The reader must proceed through Modules 1 (Basics of Mycology) and 2 (Laboratory Procedures for Fungal Culture and Isolation) and then study the remaining units, depending on his or her area of particular interest.

MEK

Acknowledgments

There are many wonderful people whose help made this text possible. William J. Rauch, DA, of Westat edited the manuscript of the second edition and helped with computer printouts.

The personnel of the mycology laboratories at Walter Reed Army Medical Center and The University Hospitals and Veterans Affairs Medical Center in Oklahoma City, in particular Kerry Snow, BS, MT(ASCP), Arthur Guruswamy, SM(ASCP), and Dayl J. Flournoy, PhD, were extremely generous with their supplies, cultures, equipment, reference materials, and good advice.

Thanks as well to the text readers and reviewers (list of reviewers follows) for their constuctive comments. We are also grateful to the various publishing companies and authors for giving permission to reproduce their photographs and charts in the book.

Acknowledgment must definitely be given to the staff at F. A. Davis, especially Jean-François Vilain, Publisher, Allied Health; Crystal Spraggins, Developmental Editor; Herbert Powell, Jr., Manager of Production; Robert C. Butler, Production Manager; Rose Gabbay, Editorial Manager; and Jessica Howie Martin, Production Editor. They did a superb job of encouraging our efforts and coordinating the text with numerous charts, drawings, and photographs.

Most of all, we thank our families—Bill Rauch, Carrie Singer, Kelly Singer, W. Lee Blevins, and Aimee Blevins—for their patience and support during the many months spent preparing the manuscript for the second edition.

MEK
KSB

Reviewers

Patricia Collins, MS, MT(ASCP)SM
Center for Rural Health
University of Kentucky
Hazard, Kentucky

Daniel P. deRegnier, MS, MT(ASCP)
Assistant Professor
Clinical Laboratory Sciences
College of Allied Health Sciences
Ferris State University
Big Rapids, Michigan

Karen S. Long, MS, CLS(NCA), MT(ASCP)
Associate Professor
Medical Technology Program
West Virginia University
Morgantown, West Virginia

Anne T. Rodgers, PhD, MT(ASCP), CLS(NCA)
Associate Professor of Medical Technology
Armstrong Atlantic State University
Savannah, Georgia

Susan B. Roman, MMSc, MT(ASCP)SM
Assistant Professor
Department of Nutrition and Laboratory Technologies
School of Allied Health Professions
College of Health Sciences
Georgia State University
Atlanta, Georgia

Contents

MODULE 2 Laboratory Procedures for Fungal Culture and Isolation — 27

MODULE 3 Common Fungal Opportunists — 73

MODULE 4 Superficial and Dermatophytic Fungi 115

MODULE 5 Yeasts 143

MODULE 6 Organisms Causing Subcutaneous Mycoses 165

MODULE 7 Organisms Causing Systemic Mycoses   193

List of Techniques and Procedures

List of Charts

MODULE 5 Yeasts

MODULE 6 Organisms Causing Subcutaneous Mycoses

MODULE 7 Organisms Causing Systemic Mycoses

List of Color Plates*

*Please note: Most of these photographs are of fungi growing on Sabouraud dextrose agar. Although SABHI agar is suggested in this second edition, colonial morphology between the two growth media is similar.

Introduction: How to Use This Text

Medical Mycology: A Self-Instrucional Text was written specifically for the beginning student of mycology. The more common fungi and funguslike bacteria encountered in a medical laboratory are well represented, with emphasis on subtle differences between similar-appearing organisms. This text will be useful for reaching a final identification in most situations. However, comprehensive books on the subject should always be maintained for those instances when more detailed information is required, for example, in speciating unusual strains of *Aspergillus*.

This text is written in a self-teaching context; to receive the most benefit from it, be sure to read the prerequisites, behavioral objectives, and content outline at the front of each module before delving into the main body of the chapter. The prerequisites stress a good microbiology background and completion of Modules 1 and 2. The intent is to provide a thorough understanding of basic terms and techniques, so that vocabulary used in succeeding chapters will be familiar. The objectives are vital; besides supplying important points to consider while reading through the text, they present ways to correlate various pieces of information. Objectives also aid in correctly answering study questions interspersed in the chapter. A content outline is provided, which shows how each topic fits into the overall picture. This is especially useful in Module 1, where the large number of new terms may be confusing if not kept in perspective.

Upon examining the main portion of each chapter, look up the charts, photos, drawings and so forth referred to in the text. Usually the chart or figure is located very close to the first place of mention, but color photographs are all in the back of the book. Much essential information is contained in these learning aids, and if they are carefully studied, a more complete comprehension of the subject will be attained. New words are in boldface when initially used, and the definition follows the term. These terms may also be found in the Glossary (Appendix C). Since mycology has undergone many nomenclature changes recently, old fungal genera and diseases are in parentheses behind the new ones. Appendix B provides a list of synonyms and currently accepted names. Recipes and procedures are highlighted in gray boxes, following the appropriate test discussions. In this manner, formulas do not clutter up the text, yet all information regarding each test is in one vicinity.

After reading each module section, quiz your retention and understanding by completing the study questions; these will identify weak areas that require further concentration. Look up the answers in Appendix A, and correctly complete any missed questions before proceeding. At the end of each module is a final exam, which should be worked in the same way. Some chapters continue with topics such as DNA testing, culture preservation, therapy for mycoses, serology, and disease descriptions. They are followed by study questions that incorporate information from the entire module.

Although mycology can be complex, it is fascinating if understood. It is hoped that this book will contribute toward that end.

Basics of Mycology

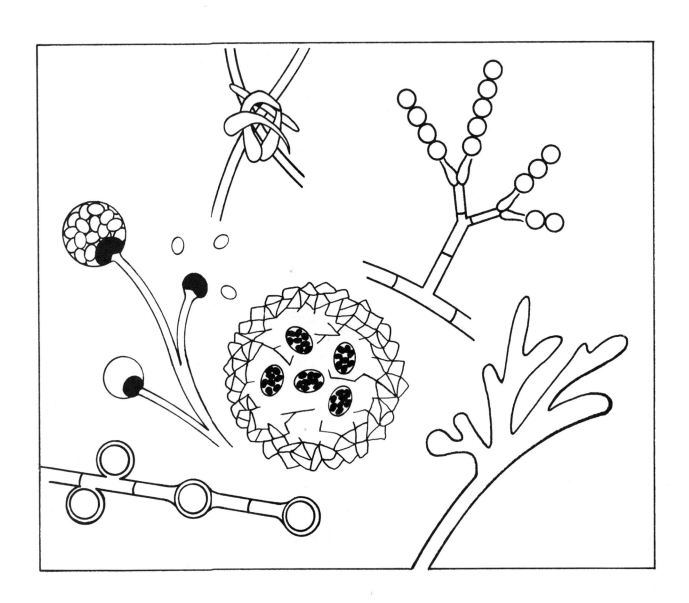

Basics of Mycology

PREREQUISITES

The learner must possess a good background knowledge in clinical microbiology.

BEHAVIORAL OBJECTIVES

Upon completion of this module, the learner should be able to:

1 Correctly recognize, from fungal cultures, photographs, or drawings:

Hyphae	Phialide
Mycelium	Phialoconidium
Aseptate hyphae	Sporangiospore
Septate hyphae	Sporangiophore
Vegetative hyphae	Sporangium
Aerial hyphae	Columella
Favic chandeliers	Ascospore
Nodular organs	Ascus
Racquet hyphae	Ascocarp
Spiral hyphae	Cleistothecium
Yeasts	Basidiospore
Arthroconidia	Basidium
Blastoconidia	Zygospore
Pseudohyphae	Cottony texture
Chlamydoconidia	Velvety texture
Annellide	Granular texture
Annelloconidium	Glabrous texture
Macro/microconidia	Rugose topography
Poroconidium	Umbonate topography
Conidiophore	Verrucose topography

2 Define:

Fungus	
Mycology	Superficial mycosis
Dimorphism	Cutaneous mycosis
Conidiogenous	Subcutaneous mycosis
Sessile	Systemic mycosis
Intercalary	Anamorph
Terminal	Teleomorph

3 Given a fungal culture, accurately describe its texture, topography, and front and reverse color.

4 Given the sexual reproduction of a fungus, discuss its taxonomy, including possible types of asexual reproduction, hyphal septation, and two medically important representative genera.

5 State whether infected material from a specific body site represents a superficial, cutaneous, subcutaneous, or systemic mycosis.

6 Given a fungal structure, state if it is reproductive or nonreproductive, and if it is the former, briefly describe how it reproduces.

CONTENT OUTLINE

I. Introduction
II. Microscopic morphology
   A. General information
      1. Hyphae
         a. Aseptate hyphae
         b. Septate hyphae
         c. Vegetative versus aerial hyphae
         d. Nonreproductive vegetative hyphae
            (1) Favic chandeliers
            (2) Nodular organs
            (3) Racquet hyphae
            (4) Spiral hyphae
      2. Yeasts
      3. Dimorphism
      4. Study questions
   B. Reproduction
      1. Asexual reproduction
         a. Conidia
            (1) Blastoconidia
            (2) Poroconidia
            (3) Phialoconidia
            (4) Annelloconidia
            (5) Macroconidia
            (6) Chlamydoconidia
            (7) Arthroconidia
         b. Sporangiospores
         c. Study questions
      2. Sexual reproduction
         a. Ascospores
         b. Basidiospores
         c. Zygospores
III. Colonial morphology
   A. Texture
      1. Cottony or woolly texture
      2. Velvety texture
      3. Granular or powdery texture
      4. Glabrous texture
   B. Topography
      1. Rugose topography
      2. Umbonate topography
      3. Verrucose topography
   C. Color
IV. Taxonomy
V. Types of mycoses based on body site
VI. Final exam

FOLLOW-UP ACTIVITIES

1 Students may observe fungal colonies and microscopic preparations and identify various structures in each.
2 Students may perform a literature search to find the taxonomic classification schemes that have enjoyed prominence in the last 10 years.

REFERENCES

Ainsworth, GC: The Fungi, Vol. IV B. Academic Press, New York, 1979.

Alexopoulos, CJ and Mims, CW: Introductory Mycology, ed 3. John Wiley & Sons, New York, 1979.

Beneke, ES and Rogers, AL: Medical Mycology Manual, ed 4. Burgess Publishing Co., Minneapolis, 1980.

Cole, GT and Samson, RA: Patterns of Development in Conidial Fungi. Pitman Publishing, London, 1978.

Kwon-Chung, KJ and Bennett J: Medical Mycology, Lea & Febiger, Philadelphia, 1992.

McGinnis, MR: Laboratory Handbook of Medical Mycology. Academic Press, New York, 1981.

Ross, IK: Biology of the Fungi. McGraw-Hill, New York, 1979.

INTRODUCTION In order to be a successful cook, you must know the names of ingredients and utensils. In order to learn medical mycology, you must of course be familiar with the vocabulary. This module presents the basic terminology used in medical mycology, as well as various forms of reproduction observed in fungi. As you follow through this module, refer to the content outline to get a clearer idea of how each item fits into the whole.

Mycology is the study of **fungi,** which are organisms that contain true nuclei (are eukaryotic), are devoid of chlorophyll, and absorb all nutrients from the environment, especially from decaying organic matter. Fungi are observed in two ways: under the microscope (microscopically) and as a colony on an agar plate (macroscopically).

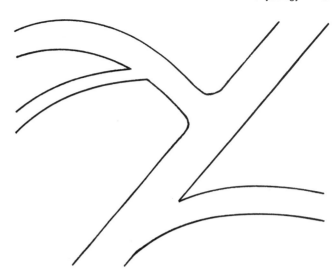

Figure 1–1. Aseptate hyphae.

MICROSCOPIC MORPHOLOGY

GENERAL INFORMATION

Microscopically, fungal cells are observed either as hyphae (molds) or as yeasts.

Hyphae

Aseptate Hyphae (Fig. 1–1)

Hyphae may be **aseptate,** meaning they have no cross walls, as in the taxonomic phylum Zygomycota. In the past, the point was often overlooked that zygomycetous organisms are *usually* aseptate rather than completely so: cross walls may be evident at damaged areas and near reproductive structures. These hyphae are wide and ribbonlike, measuring 6 to 10 μm in diameter.

Septate Hyphae (Fig. 1–2)

Most hyphae are **septate,** with cell cross walls very evident, as in the phyla Ascomycota, Basidiomycota, and Deuteromycota. These hyphae are 3 to 4 μm in diameter. For the taxonomic classification, see the later section of this module.

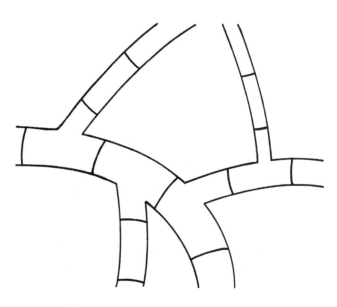

Figure 1–2. Septate hyphae.

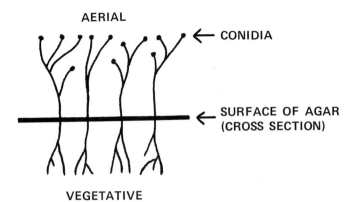

AERIAL

← CONIDIA

← SURFACE OF AGAR
(CROSS SECTION)

VEGETATIVE

Figure 1–3. Cross view—vegetative and aerial hyphae.

Vegetative versus Aerial Hyphae (Fig. 1–3)

In a cross-section of a mold culture, the **vegetative,** or food-absorbing, portion of the mycelium is under the surface of the agar. The **aerial** hyphae extend above the agar surface and may support reproductive structures, commonly called conidia, at their tips. Color Plates 1 and 2 (see back of book) show the distinct color differences sometimes observed between the aerial hyphae, on the front side of the colony, and the vegetative hyphae, on the reverse side.

Nonreproductive Vegetative Hyphae

Vegetative hyphae may possess some very distinct nonreproductive characteristics, which may aid in speciation.

Favic Chandeliers (Figs. 1–4 and 1–5)

Favic chandeliers resemble the antlers of a buck deer, with the ends of the hyphae blunt and branched. Favic chandeliers are diagnostic for identifying cultures of *Trichophyton schoenleinii,* an organism that causes **dermatophytosis**(ringworm of skin, hair, or nail).

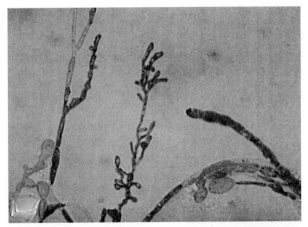

Figure 1–4. Favic chandeliers, *Trichophyton schoenleinii,* lactophenol cotton blue (LPCB) stain (magnification ×450).

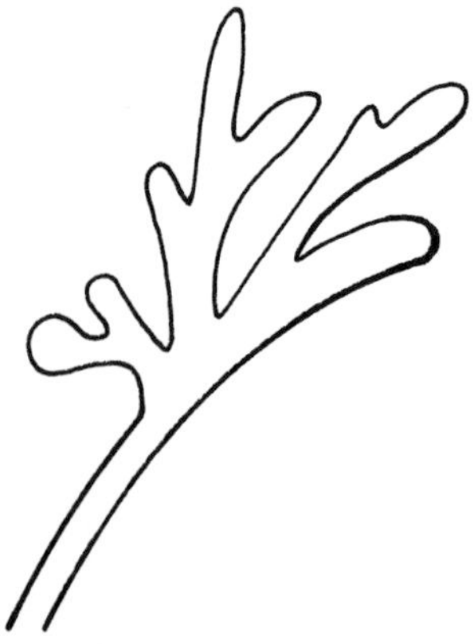

Figure 1–5. Favic chandeliers.

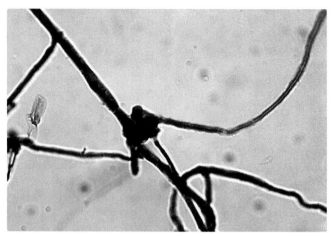

Figure 1–6. Nodular organ, *Microsporum ferrugineum*, LPCB stain (magnification ×450).

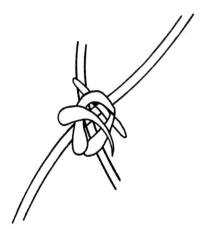

Figure 1–7. Nodular organ.

Nodular Organs (Figs. 1–6 and 1–7)
Nodular organs are knots of twisted hyphae.

Racquet Hyphae (Figs. 1–8 and 1–9)
The name **racquet hyphae** is given because the hyphae resemble tennis racquets placed end to end.

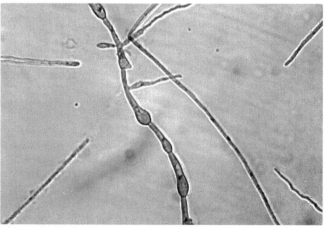

Figure 1–8. Racquet hyphae, *Trichophyton ajelloi*, LPCB stain (magnification ×450).

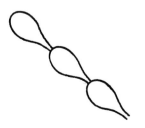

Figure 1–9. Racquet hyphae.

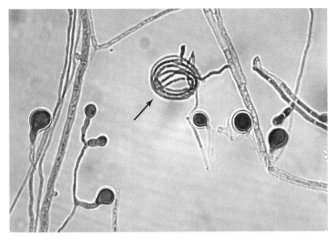

Figure 1–10. Spiral hyphae (arrow) *Chrysosporium* sp., LPCB stain (magnification × 450).

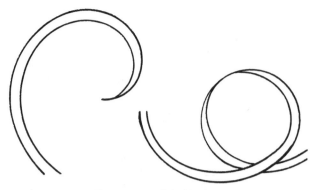

Figure 1–11. Spiral hyphae.

Spiral Hyphae (Figs. 1–10 and 1–11)

Spiral hyphae may be flat or may turn like a corkscrew. They are commonly observed in older cultures.

Yeasts (Fig. 1–12)   **Yeasts** consist of individual oval to round cells, which frequently bud to form daughter cells.

Dimorphism   Most fungi exist only as molds or as yeasts. Some fungi, however, may exhibit **dimorphism,** meaning that they possess two distinct phases. At room temperature (25 or 30°C) they grow as molds (mold phase); at body temperature (37°C) or incubator temperature (35°C), they change and grow as yeasts (yeast or tissue phase). Conversion from one form to the other is one of the primary aids in identifying these fungi. Most of the dimorphic organisms produce serious and often fatal systemic diseases.

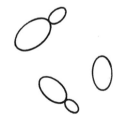

Figure 1–12. Budding yeasts.

STUDY QUESTIONS

1. Circle true or false:

   T   F   Fungi resemble plants in that both contain chlorophyll.

2. A patient's sputum specimen contains a dimorphic fungus. If the sputum is put on a slide and a coverslip added, what would you expect to observe—hyphae or yeasts?

3. Circle the correct answer:
   Knots of twisted hyphae are called conidia/nodular organs.

4. Circle the letter of the correct answer:
   Figure 1–13 is a drawing of:
   A. Racquet hyphae

   B. Nodular organs

   C. Yeasts

   D. Favic chandeliers

   E. Aerial hyphae

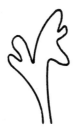

Figure 1–13. Study question demonstration.

STOP HERE UNTIL YOU HAVE COMPLETED THE ANSWERS.

Look up the answers in the back of the book. If you missed more than two of them, go back and review the General Information section. Correctly complete any missed questions.

REPRODUCTION

Fungi exhibit just about every type of reproduction. They multiply both asexually and sexually. Depending on the circumstances, fungi may use more than one of these methods to multiply.

Asexual Reproduction

Asexual reproduction is so called because there is merely nuclear and cytoplasmic division, or mitosis, just as with normally growing, nonreproducing cells. **Sexual reproduction** involves fusion of two nuclei into a zygote.

Conidia (Singular, Conidium)

The field of **conidiogenesis,** or asexual (anamorph) conidium formation, has undergone dramatic changes in the last decade, and the vocabulary has become very complicated and confusing. At present, fungi are classified by this ontogeny, so some of the more important terms must be reviewed. Chart 1–1 sums up the essentials. **Conidia** may originate **blastically,** meaning the **conidiogenous** (parent) cell enlarges, then a septum separates the enlarged portion into a daughter cell. Or they may develop **thallically,** in which a septum forms first, and the growing point ahead of it becomes the daughter. The prefix **holo** in front of these words indicates that all wall layers of the parent cell are involved in daughter conidium development, while the prefix **entero** means that only the inner cell wall layers are included. **Arthric** conidiogenesis is a subheading under thallic; arthric daughter cells fragment within the hyphal strand before dispersing.

CHART 1-1. CONIDIOGENESIS*

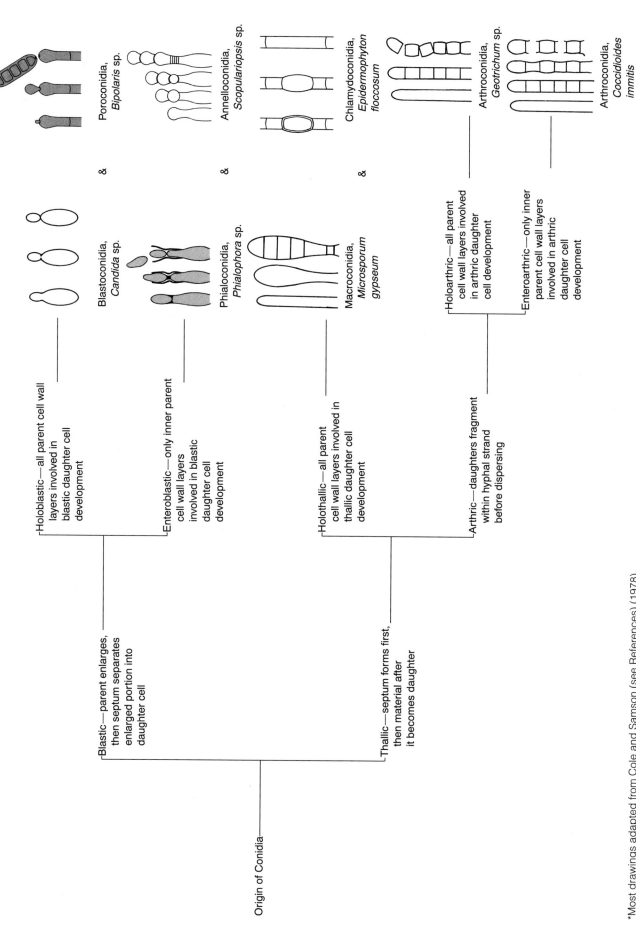

Origin of Conidia

Blastic—parent enlarges, then septum separates enlarged portion into daughter cell

Holoblastic—all parent cell wall layers involved in blastic daughter cell development

Blastoconidia, *Candida* sp.

Poroconidia, *Bipolaris* sp.

&

Annelloconidia, *Scopulariopsis* sp.

Enteroblastic—only inner parent cell wall layers involved in blastic daughter cell development

Phialoconidia, *Phialophora* sp.

Chlamydoconidia, *Epidermophyton floccosum*

Thallic—septum forms first, then material after it becomes daughter

Holothallic—all parent cell wall layers involved in thallic daughter cell development

Macroconidia, *Microsporum gypseum*

&

Arthric—daughters fragment within hyphal strand before dispersing

Holoarthric—all parent cell wall layers involved in arthric daughter cell development

Arthroconidia, *Geotrichum* sp.

&

Enteroarthric—only inner parent cell wall layers involved in arthric daughter cell development

Arthroconidia, *Coccidioides immitis*

*Most drawings adapted from Cole and Samson (see References) (1978)

11

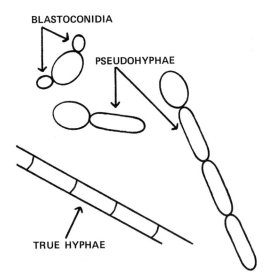

Figure 1–14. Blastoconidia, pseudohyphae, and true hyphae.

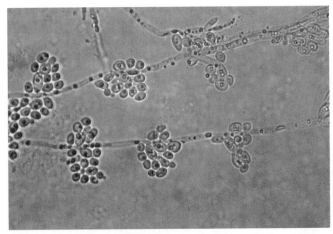

Figure 1–15. Blastoconidia and pseudohyphae, *Candida albicans* (magnification × 450).

Blastoconidia (Blastospores) (Figs. 1–14 and 1–15)
Blastoconidia, produced by budding, may be seen in molds, such as *Cladosporium,* or in yeasts, such as *Candida.* In some yeast species, these blastoconidia elongate to form **pseudohyphae,** which often align end to end (Fig. 1–15). Pseudohyphae may be differentiated from true hyphae in that the cells of the former are constricted at their points of attachment (see Fig. 1–14).

Poroconidia (Fig. 1–16)
Poroconidia, seen in *Bipolaris,* are formed by the daughter pushing through a minute pore in the parent cell. The parent may be in a long stalk **(conidiophore),** or it may be a specialized conidiogenous cell.

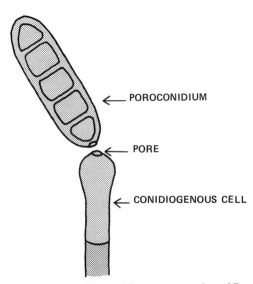

Figure 1–16. Poroconidium, pore, and conidiogenous cell.

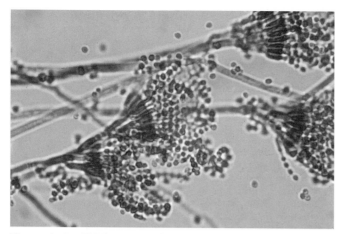

Figure 1–17. Phialides and phialoconidia on elaborate branching conidiophores, *Penicillin* sp., LPCB stain (magnification ×450).

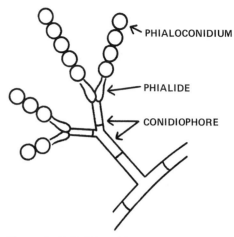

Figure 1–18. Phialoconidium, phialide, and conidiophore.

Phialoconidia (Figs. 1–17 and 1–18)

Phialoconidia, elicited from a tube- or vase-shaped conidiogenous structure termed a **phialide,** may be illustrated in *Penicillium.* The first phialoconidium is holoblastic, but the rest develop enteroblastically. In *Penicillium* (Fig. 1–17) and *Aspergillus,* the phialides were formerly called sterigmata; this old word is now reserved for organisms in the taxonomic phylum Basidiomycota. Phialides may exhibit a terminal cup-shaped **collarette.** The supporting conidiophore may be simple or it may be elaborately branched (Fig. 1–18).

Annelloconidia (Fig. 1–19)

Annelloconidia, observed in *Scopulariopsis,* are grown from inside a vase-shaped conidiogenous **annellide.** The first annelloconidium is holoblastic, while the rest are enteroblastic. As each conidium is released, a ring of parent outer cell wall material remains behind, giving a distinct saw-toothed appearance to the sides of the annellide. The supporting structure is termed an **annellophore,** and it may be simple or it may be elaborately branched (Fig. 1–19).

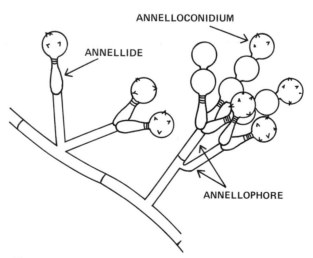

Figure 1–19. Annelloconidium, annellide, and annellophores.

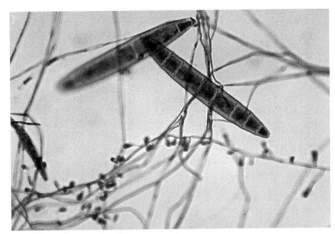

Figure 1–20. Macroconidia and microconidia, *Microsporum vanbreuseghemii*, LPCB stain (magnification ×450).

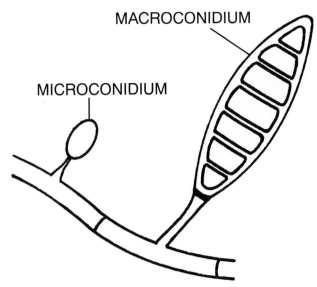

Figure 1–21. Macroconidium and microconidium.

Macroconidia (Figs. 1–20 and 1–21)

A **macroconidium** (macroaleuriospore) arises by conversion of an entire hyphal element into a multicelled conidium. A **microconidium** (microaleuriospore) is produced in the same manner, except the new conidium remains aseptate. The terms macroconidia and microconidia are not used unless both types are apparent in the same culture, when there is a need to differentiate them. Macroconidia may be thick- or thin-walled, spiny or smooth, and club-shaped or oval. They may be **sessile,** arising on the sides of the hyphae, or supported by conidiophores, and they are observed individually or in clusters. Microconidia are usually one celled and round, oval, or club-shaped. They may be sessile or supported alone or in clusters by a conidiophore.

Chlamydoconidia (Figs. 1–22, 1–23, and 1–24)

Chlamydoconidia, thick-walled survival conidia formed during unpleasant environmental conditions, will germinate and produce conidia when a better climate occurs. They may be observed at the hyphal tip **(terminal),** on the sides **(sessile),** or within the hyphal strand **(intercalary).**

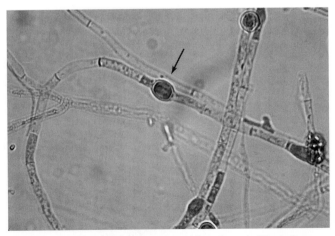

Figure 1–22. Intercalary chlamydoconidium (arrow) *Gliocladium* sp., LPCB stain (magnification ×450).

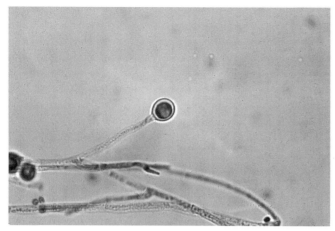

Figure 1–23. Terminal chlamydoconidium, *Gliocladium* sp., LPCB stain (magnification ×450).

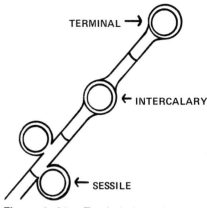

Figure 1–24. Terminal, intercalary, and sessile chlamydoconidia.

In the past, these structures were termed chlamydospores, and they were grouped together with the similar-appearing forms seen in yeasts such as *Candida albicans*. However, the yeast **chlamydospores** are thick-walled vesicles and not conidia, since they neither germinate nor produce conidia when mature. In this text, yeast vesicles will be called chlamydospores, while the word chlamydoconidia applies to germinating structures.

Arthroconidia (Arthrospores) (Figs. 1–25 and 1–26)
Arthroconidia (Fig. 1–25) fragment from the hyphae through the septation points. They separate within the parent hyphal strand before dispersing. Arthroconidia may form adjacent to each other within the hyphae, or they may be separated by alternating empty spaces, **disjunctor cells,** giving a checkered appearance. It is important to determine if the arthroconidia are adjacent or alternate, as *Coccidioides immitis* is partly identified by the presence of disjunctor cells. Arthroconidia mature to be thick-walled and barrel-shaped or rectangular (Fig. 1–26).

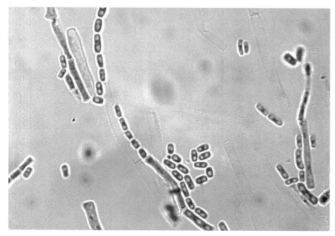

Figure 1–25. Arthroconidia, *Geotrichum candidum*, LPCB stain (magnification ×450).

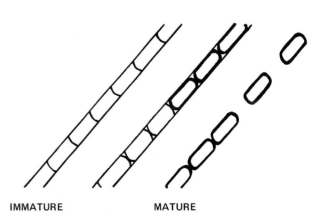

IMMATURE   MATURE

Figure 1–26. Arthroconidia.

Sporangiospores (Figs. 1–27 and 1–28)

Sporangiospores are separate from conidia because they are only formed in aseptate fungi, whereas conidia are only formed in septate fungi. Sporangiospores are formed by internal cleavage of the contents of a sac called a **sporangium** (plural, sporangia). The sporangium is supported on a base, or **columella,** and it in turn is supported by a stalk-like **sporangiophore.** New sporangia may be empty, while older ones are filled with spores. When the sporangium dissolves and disperses its contents, the columella remains. Sporangiospores are only observed in the taxonomic phylum Zygomycota.

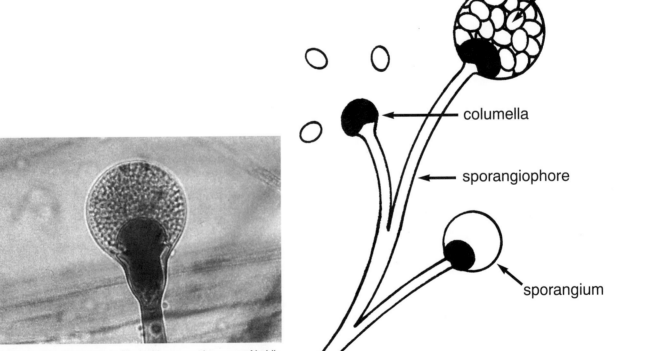

Figure 1–27. Sporangium filled with sporangiospores, *Absidia* sp., LPCB stain (magnification ×450).

Figure 1–28. Sporangia containing a columella and sporangiospores.

STUDY QUESTIONS

1. See Figure 1–29. What type of reproductive structure is observed? Circle the letter of the correct answer:
   A. Macroconidium
   B. Phialoconidium
   C. Microconidium
   D. Sporangiospore
   E. Blastoconidium

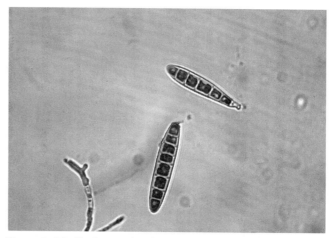

Figure 1–29. Study question demonstration, LPCB stain (magnification ×450).

2. Circle true or false:
   T F   Arthroconidia reproduce by fragmentation.

3. Circle true or false:
   T F   Chlamydospores of *Candida albicans* will germinate to form new conidia when mature.

4. Circle the letter of the correct answer. The conidiogenous cell in Figure 1–30 is a(an):
   A. Phialide
   B. Sporangium
   C. Poroconidium
   D. Annellide
   E. Chlamydoconidium

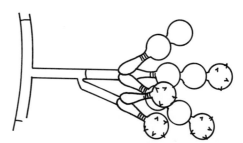

Figure 1–30. Study question demonstration.

5. Circle the letter of the correct answer. Blastoconidia that have elongated are termed:

   A. Mother cells

   B. True hyphae

   C. Chlamydospores

   D. Conidia

   E. Pseudohyphae

6. From Figure 1–31, fill in the blanks:

   A. _____

   B. _____

   C. _____

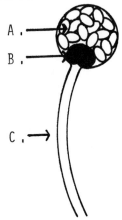

Figure 1–31. Study question demonstration.

STOP HERE UNTIL YOU HAVE COMPLETED THE ANSWERS.

Look up the answers in the back of the book. If you missed more than one, go back and repeat the section on asexual reproduction. Correctly complete any missed questions before proceeding

---

Sexual Reproduction   Those fungi that have a sexual or teleomorph stage are called the **Perfect Fungi.** Those whose sexual stage does not exist or has not yet been discovered are in the taxonomic phylum Deuteromycota, or **Fungi Imperfecti.** The commonly observed sexual mechanisms in medically important fungi follow.

Ascospores (Figs. 1–32, 1–33, and 1–34)

The nucleus from a male cell, called an **antheridium,** passes through a bridge into the female cell, an **ascogonium.** The male and female cells may be from the same, self-compatible colony or from two colonies of opposite mating types. Once the male and female

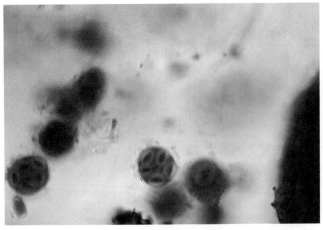

Figure 1–32. Ascus with ascopores, *Aspergillus* sp., LPCB stain (magnification × 1000).

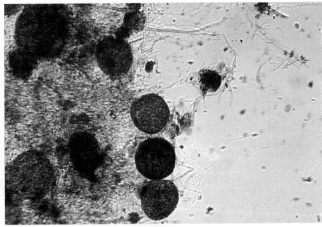

Figure 1–33. Cleistothecia, *Aspergillus* sp., LPCB stain (magnification × 100).

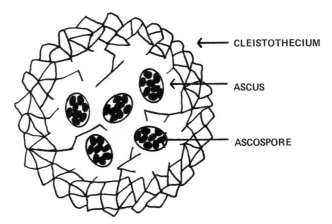

Figure 1–34. Cleistothecium, ascus, and ascospore.

nuclei fuse to form a **zygote,** the cell becomes an **ascus** (plural, asci). The diploid zygote nucleus divides by meiosis to form four haploid nuclei, which in turn divide by mitosis to form eight nuclei. Each new nucleus walls off inside the ascus to form an **ascospore.**

Some ascomycetous fungi, for example, the yeast *Saccharomyces cerevisiae,* exhibit unprotected asci, whereas others, for example, the mold *Pseudallescheria boydii* produce asci within a somatic saclike structure called an **ascocarp.** The ascocarp observed in medically important fungi is completely enclosed and is termed a **cleistothecium.** Ascospores are formed by the phylum Ascomycota.

Basidiospores (Fig. 1–35)
A binucleate mycelium is formed by fusion of two compatible hyphae or yeast cells, usually with the aid of clamp connections:

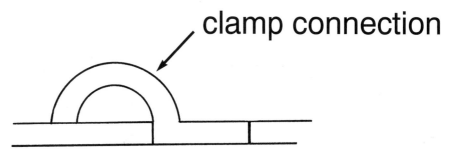

The terminal cell of the resulting mycelium enlarges into a club-shaped structure called a **basidium.** The two nuclei within the basidium fuse to form a zygote, then undergo meiosis to produce four haploid nuclei. Four little protrusions (**basidiospores**) (Fig. 1–35) extend out from the end of the basidium, and each haploid nucleus travels

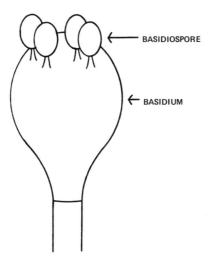

Figure 1–35. Basidiospore and basidium.

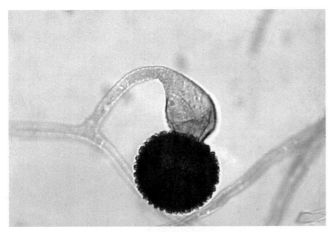

Figure 1–36. Zygosporangium, *Zygorhynchus* sp., LPCB stain (magnification ×450).

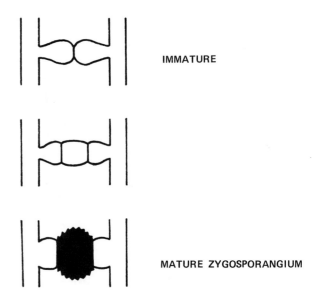

IMMATURE

MATURE ZYGOSPORANGIUM

Figure 1–37. Zygosporangium.

into a basidiospore. Some Basidiomycetes, such as mushrooms, produce a protective **basidiocarp** to lodge the basidia and basidiospores. The only really important Basidiomycete in medical mycology is *Filobasidiella neoformans*, the sexual stage of *Cryptococcus neoformans*. Basidiospores are formed by the phylum Basidiomycota.

Zygospores (Figs. 1–36 and 1–37)
Two compatible hyphae each form an arm **(zygophore)** extending toward the other. The hyphae may be from a self-compatible colony or from two colonies of opposite mating types. When the zygophores meet, they fuse to form a thick-walled, protective **zygosporangium** (Figs. 1–36 and 1–37) within which a **zygospore** develops. Zygospores are formed by the taxonomic phylum Zygomycota.

COLONIAL MORPHOLOGY

Although many fungi do not have a colonial morphology characteristic enough to allow identification without additional criteria, some are very distinct. Certain general terms are used to describe fungal colonies.

TEXTURE (Fig. 1–38)

The colonial **texture** describes the height of the aerial hyphae. The textural terms are relative and are best described in a cross-sectional drawing (Fig. 1–38).

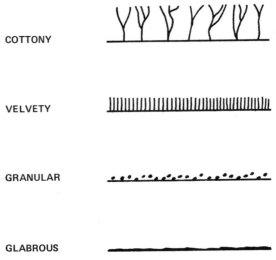

COTTONY

VELVETY

GRANULAR

GLABROUS

Figure 1–38. Colonial textures.

Cottony or Woolly Texture **Cottony** or **woolly** colonies produce a very high, dense aerial mycelium (see Color Plate 3).

Velvety Texture **Velvety** colonies produce a low aerial mycelium which resembles the fabric velvet (see Color Plate 4).

Granular or Powdery Texture **Granular** or **powdery** colonies are flat and crumbly because of the dense production of conidia. The granular texture is rougher, like granulated sugar, and the powdery texture is like flour (see Color Plate 5). These two terms are often used interchangeably.

Glabrous Texture **Glabrous** or **waxy** colonies have a smooth surface because they produce no aerial mycelium (see Color Plate 6). Usually yeasts form a glabrous macroscopic appearance.

TOPOGRAPHY (Fig. 1–39) Colonial **topography** describes the various designs of hills and valleys seen on fungal cultures. The topography is often masked by the aerial hyphae; therefore, this characteristic is better observed on the reverse side of the colony. A colony may possess no topography; that is, it is flat.

Rugose Topography **Rugose** colonies have deep furrows irregularly radiating from the center of the culture (see Color Plate 7).

Umbonate Topography **Umbonate** colonies possess a buttonlike central elevation. They may be accompanied by rugose furrows around the button (see Color Plate 8).

Verrucose Topography **Verrucose** colonies exhibit a wrinkled, convoluted surface (see Color Plate 9).

COLOR Be as specific about the colony colors as possible. For example, instead of describing a culture as brown, use words such as beige, tan, khaki, or mahogany. If there are concentric rings of different colors, observe each one. Be sure to characterize both the front and reverse sides of the culture.

TAXONOMY The taxonomy of fungi has undergone very rapid changes in the last several years, and there is no general agreement yet on an ultimate classification schema. Organisms are classified by their sexual (teleomorph) stage. Organisms with no known sexual stage are classified in the phylum Deuteromycota. See Chart 1–2. Fungi in parentheses represent the asexual (anamorph) name. Those without parentheses indicate

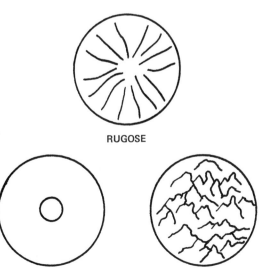

Figure 1–39. Colonial topographies.

RUGOSE

UMBONATE VERRUCOSE

CHART 1–2. TAXONOMIC CLASSIFICATION OF CLINICALLY IMPORTANT FUNGI AND FUNGUSLIKE BACTERIA*

Representative Genera	Asexual Reproduction	Sexual Reproduction	Hyphae
TRUE FUNGI: Kingdom Myceteae (Fungi)			

Phylum Zygomycota
Class Zygomycetes
Order Mucorales
  Family Mucoraceae—*Absidia, Mucor, Rhizopus, Circinella*
  Family Cunninghamellaceae—*Cunninghamella*
  Family Syncephalastraceae—*Syncephalastrum*
  Family Mortierellaceae—*Mortierella*
	Sporangiospores, sometimes chlamydoconidia or budding	Zygospores	6–10 μm in diameter, usually aseptate, except at bases of reproductive structures or across damaged areas

Phylum Ascomycota
Class Ascomycetes
Subclass Hemiascomycetidae
Order Endomycetales
  Family Endomycetaceae—*Endomyces (Geotrichum)*
  Family Saccharomycetaceae—*Saccharomyces*
Subclass Plectomycetidae
Order Onygenales
  Family Gymnoascaceae—*Arthroderma (Trichophyton), Nannizzia (Microsporum), Ajellomyces (Blastomyces, Histoplasma)*
Order Eurotiales
  Family Eurotiaceae—*Talaromyces, Eupenicillium (Penicillium); Eurotium, Sartorya, Emericella (Aspergillus); Byssochlamys (Paecilomyces)*
Subclass Loculoascomycetidae
Order Myriangiales
  Family Saccardinulaceae—*Piedraia*
	Fission, fragmentation, chlamydoconidia, conidia	Ascospores	3–4 μm in diameter, septate

Classification	Sexual spores	Asexual spores	Size
Phylum Basidiomycota Class Basidiomycetes Subclass Teliomycetidae Order Ustilaginales Family Ustilaginaceae—*Filobasidium, Filobasidiella (Cryptococcus); Rhodosporidium (Rhodotorula)*	Basidiospores	Budding, arthroconidia, conidia, oidia, mycelial fragmentation	3–4 μm in diameter, septate
Phylum Deuteromycota Form—Class Blastomycetes Form—Order Sporobolomycetales—*(Sporobolomyces)* Form—Order Cryptococcales—*(Rhodotorula), (Cryptococcus), (Candida), (Trichosporon), (Malassezia)* Form—Class Coelomycetes Form—Order Sphaeropsidales Form—Family Sphaeropsidaceae—*(Phoma), (Sphaeropsis)* Form—Class Hyphomycetes Form—Order Moniliales Form—Family Moniliaceae—*(Aspergillus), (Penicillium), (Botrytis), (Verticillium), (Trichoderma), (Paracoccidioides), (Sporothrix), (Geotrichum), (Coccidioides), (Microsporum), (Trichophyton), (Epidermophyton), (Acremonium), (Paecilomyces)* Form—Family Dematiaceae—*(Alternaria), (Curvularia), (Bipolaris), (Cladosporium), (Phialophora), (Fonsecaea), (Exophiala), (Wangiella)* Form—Family Tuberculariaceae—*(Volutella), (Fusarium)*	None or not yet discovered	Conidia	3–4 μm in diameter, septate
FUNGUSLIKE BACTERIA: Kingdom Monera (Bacteria) Phylum Schizomycota Order Actinomycetales Family Mycobacteriaceae Family Actinomycetaceae—*Actinomyces, Nocardia* Family Streptomycetaceae—*Streptomyces*			0.5–1.0 μm in diameter

* Sexual names are without parentheses. Corresponding asexual names are in parentheses adjacent to the matching sexual name.

the sexual (**teleomorph**) name. For example, *Filobasidiella* is the sexual name, and *Cryptococcus* is the asexual name. Some asexual fungi may exhibit two or three different sexual appearances and thus may possess two or three different sexual names. The reverse is also true: some sexual organisms may possess two or three different asexual names.

TYPES OF MYCOSES BASED ON BODY SITE

Mycoses, fungal diseases, may be classified according to the tissue or body site invaded.

Superficial mycoses affect only the outermost layers of skin and hair. Little or no pathology is evidenced, and the patients are mainly worried about cosmetic effects. Some superficial mycoses are otomycosis, black and white piedra, pityriasis versicolor, and tinea nigra.

Cutaneous mycoses involve destruction of the keratin of skin, hair, and nails. There is rarely invasion of deeper body tissues. Cutaneous mycoses are caused primarily by the dermatophytes *(Trichophyton, Microsporum,* and *Epidermophyton)* and by *Candida.*

Subcutaneous mycoses involve the skin, muscle, and connective tissue immediately below the skin. Deeper tissue involvement is rare. Some subcutaneous mycoses are chromoblastomycosis, mycetoma, and sporotrichosis.

Systemic mycoses involve the deep tissues and organs of the body. In disseminated forms of these diseases, subcutaneous and cutaneous areas may also be invaded. Some systemic mycoses are blastomycosis, paracoccidioidomycosis, histoplasmosis, and coccidioidomycosis.

FINAL EXAM

1. From drawings A through L, fill in the blanks:

A. _____

B. _____

C. _____

D. _____

E. _____

F. _____

G. _____

H. _____

I. _____

J. _____

K. _____

L. _____

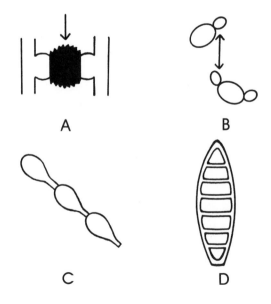

A   B

C   D

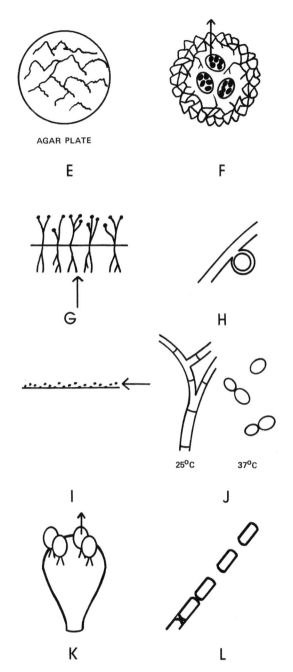

AGAR PLATE

E   F

G   H

25°C   37°C

I   J

K   L

2. See Color Plates 10 and 11. Describe the texture, topography, and front and reverse colors of this colony.

3. A patient is seen by his physician for a hard, nonmoving nodule below the skin on his right index finger. There are no other symptoms. Circle the letter of the correct answer:
   The infection that this patient is most likely presenting is:
   A. Superficial

   B. Cutaneous

   C. Subcutaneous

   D. Systemic

4. See Figure 1–40. Circle the correct answers.
   This fungus produces phialoconidia/annelloconidia. It has no known sexual stage; thus this figure must represent a(an) anamorph/teleomorph and is classified in the phylum Basidiomycota/Deuteromycota.

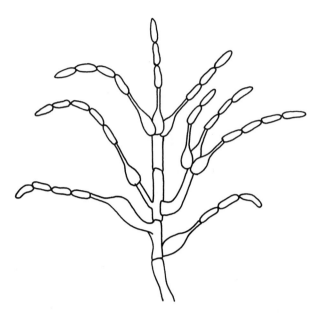

Figure 1–40. Study question demonstration.

5. In each blank, write the letter of the correct answer below.
   The taxonomic phylum Zygomycota is distinct in that the hyphae are usually _____. The typical asexual reproductive structures are _____, and the sexual stage is characterized by the formation of _____.
   A. Septate

   B. Basidiospores

   C. Zygospores

   D. Aseptate

   E. Ascospores

   F. Arthroconidia

   G. Sporangiospores

STOP HERE UNTIL YOU HAVE COMPLETED THE ANSWERS.
Look up the answers in the back of the book. If you missed more than three, go back and repeat the module. Correctly complete any missed questions.

Laboratory Procedures for Fungal Culture and Isolation

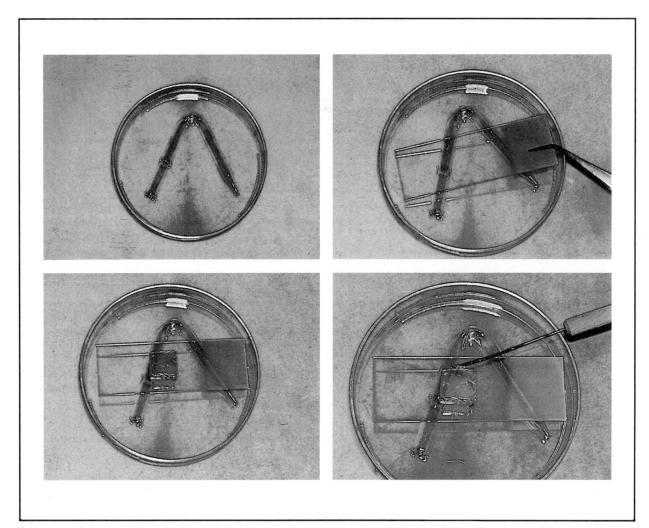

Laboratory Procedures for Fungal Culture and Isolation

PREREQUISITES

The learner must possess a good background knowledge in clinical microbiology and must have finished Module 1, Basics of Mycology.

BEHAVIORAL OBJECTIVES

Upon completion of this module, the learner should be able to:

1   List at least four general rules for good fungal specimen collection.

2   Correctly collect and process a fungal specimen from a given body source.

3   List at least two fungi which may be recovered from a given body site.

4   Explain why respiratory and urine specimens are collected in the morning, and why 24-hour collections should be avoided.

5   State two reasons why direct examination of every specimen for mycology is essential.

6   Discuss the types of specimen direct examinations, including the principle, procedure, and appearance of fungi in each.

7   Compile a rationale for use of the following primary isolation media:
SABHI
Brain heart infusion with blood (BHIB)
Sabouraud dextrose agar
Inhibitory mold agar
BHIB with gentamicin and
   chloramphenicol
BHIB with gentamicin, chloramphenicol,
   and cycloheximide

Include which medium is best for isolating a given organism and which combination of media is best for maximal fungal recovery.

8   Comment on the optimal incubation temperature(s) for primary fungal cultures and justify the reasons.

9   Define rapid, intermediate, and slow growth rates, as discussed in this module.

10   Compare and contrast the advantages and disadvantages of the tease mount, cellophane tape, slide culture, modified slide culture, and coverslip sandwich techniques for fungal examination.

11   Synthesize a fungal identification scheme, using the general criteria below:
Specimen source
Fungal growth rate
Colonial appearance
General fungal microscopic morphology
   (mold, yeast, funguslike bacterium,
   dimorphic organism)
Specific fungal microscopic morphology
   (reproductive structures and so forth)

12   List the pitfalls of skin tests for fungal infections.

13   List four immunologic methods for fungal antibody testing and fungal antigen testing, respectively.

14 List possible causes of false positive results when testing for cryptococcal antigen, and ways to decrease false positives.

15 State the principle behind the DNA probe procedure and how it is useful for fungal identification.

16 State four methods of fungal culture preservation.

17 List the five basic classes of antifungal agents and give one example of each. Discuss which mycoses (systemic disease, dermatophytes, yeasts, subcutaneous) are treated by each class of agents.

18 Discuss problems with successful antifungal treatment of immunocompromised patients.

CONTENT OUTLINE

I. Introduction
II. Obtaining and processing the specimen
   A. General considerations
      1. Collected from affected area
      2. Sterile technique in collecting specimen
      3. Adequate specimen
      4. Specimen delivered and processed quickly
      5. Specimen adequately labelled
   B. Specific fungal specimen sources
      1. Blood, bone marrow
      2. Cerebrospinal fluid
      3. Cutaneous: hair, nails, and skin
      4. Respiratory: bronchial washings, sputa, throats, transtracheal aspirates
      5. Tissue, biopsies
      6. Urine
      7. Vaginal, uterine cervix
      8. Wounds, subcutaneous lesions, mucocutaneous lesions
   C. Study questions
III. Direct examination of the specimen
   A. Saline wet preparation
   B. Lactophenol cotton blue wet mount
   C. Potassium hydroxide (KOH) preparation
   D. Gram stain
   E. Acid-fast stain
   F. India ink preparation
   G. Calcofluor white stain
   H. Other stains
   I. Study questions
IV. Culturing the specimen
   A. Primary fungal media
      1. Nonselective media
         a. Sabouraud brain heart infusion agar (SABHI)
         b. Brain heart infusion agar with blood (BHIB)
         c. Sabouraud dextrose agar (SDA)
      2. Selective media with antibiotics
         a. Inhibitory mold agar (IMA)
         b. Brain heart infusion agar with blood, gentamicin, and chloramphenicol
         c. Brain heart infusion agar with blood, gentamicin, chloramphenicol, and cycloheximide
         d. Dermatophyte test medium (DTM)
      3. Special considerations
         a. *Nocardia*
         b. *Cryptococcus neoformans* in AIDS patients
         c. *Actinomyces*
   B. Incubation temperature
   C. Incubation time
   D. Subculture media
      1. Neutral Sabouraud dextrose agar (Emmon's modification)
      2. Potato dextrose agar (PDA)
   E. Study questions
V. Examining the culture
   A. Tease mount method
   B. Cellophane tape method
   C. Slide culture method
   D. Modified slide culture method
   E. Coverslip sandwich technique
VI. Proceeding to specific modules
VII. Final examination
VIII. Supplemental rationale
   A. Skin tests
   B. Seromycology
   C. DNA testing (DNA probes and polymerase chain reaction)
   D. Culture preservation
   E. Therapy for mycoses
   F. Study questions

FOLLOW-UP ACTIVITIES

1 Students may perform direct mounts of patient specimens or fungus cultures and observe them under the microscope.

2 Students may inoculate a specific fungus onto each of the media described in this module, then compare colonial morphology, microscopic morphology, and amount of fungal growth on each medium.

3 Students may inoculate *Geotrichum candidum* onto two tubes of Sabouraud dextrose agar, incubate one tube at room temperature (25° C) and the other tube at 37° C, and then compare the two tubes for fungal growth.

4 Students may observe positive and negative reactions of the various serologic tests listed in the Supplemental Rationale section.

REFERENCES

Bretagne, S, et al: Detection of *Aspergillus* species DNA in bronchoalveolar lavage samples by competitive PCR. J Clin Microbiol 33:1164, 1995.

Camargo, ZP, et al: Monoclonal antibody capture enzyme immunoassay for detection of *Paracoccidioides brasiliensis* antibodies in paracoccidioidomycosis. J Clin Microbiol 32:2377, 1994.

Castellani, A: Further researches on the long viability and growth of many pathogenic fungi and some bacteria in sterile distilled water. Mycopath et Mycologia Applic 20:1, 1963.

Castellani, A: The viability of some pathogenic fungi in sterile distilled water. J Trop Med Hyg 42:225, 1939.

deFatima Ferreira-da-Cruz, M, et al: Sensitive immunoradiometric assay for the detection of *Paracoccidioides brasiliensis* antigens in human sera. J Clin Microbiol 29:1202, 1991.

Dewsnup, DH and Stevens, DA: Efficacy of oral amphotericin B in AIDS patients with thrush clinically resistant to fluconazole. J Med Vet Mycol 32:389, 1994.

Engler, HD and Shea, YR: Effect of potential interference factors on performance of enzyme immunoassay and latex agglutination assay for cryptococcal antigen. J Clin Microbiol 32:2307, 1994.

Friedman, GC, et al: Allergic fungal sinusitis: Report of three cases associated with dematiaceous fungi. Am J Clin Pathol Sept:368, 1991.

Fujita, SI, et al: Microtitration plate enzyme immunoassay to detect PCR-amplified DNA from *Candida* species in blood. J Clin Microbiol 33:962, 1995.

Gutierrez, J, et al: Circulating *Candida* antigens and antibodies: useful markers of candidemia. J Clin Microbiol 31:2550, 1993.

Hageage, GH and Harrington, BJ: Use of calcofluor white in clinical mycology. Lab Med 15:109, 1984.

Hamilton, J, et al: Performance of cryptococcal antigen latex agglutination kits on serum and cerebrospinal fluid specimens of AIDS patients before and after pronase treatment. J Clin Microbiol 29:333, 1991.

Harris: Modified method for fungal slide culture. J Clin Microbiol 24:460, 1986.

Heelan, J, et al: False positive reactions in the latex agglutination test for *Cryptococcus neoformans* antigen. J Clin Microbiol 29:1260, 1991.

Holmes, AR, et al: Detection of *Candida albicans* and other yeasts in blood by PCR. J Clin Microbiol 32:228, 1994.

Hopfer, RL, et al: Detection and differentiation of fungi in clinical specimens using polymerase chain reaction (PCR) amplification and restriction enzyme analysis. J Med Vet Mycol 31:65, 1993.

Huffnagle, KE and Gander, RM: Evaluation of Gen-Probe's *Histoplasma capsulatum* and *Cryptococcus neoformans* AccuProbes. J Clin Microbiol 31:419, 1993.

Kappe, R and Schulze-Berge, A: New cause for false-positive results with the Pastorex *Aspergillus* antigen latex agglutination test. J Clin Microbiol 31:2489, 1993.

Kappe, R, et al: Fluconazole in patients at risk from invasive aspergillosis. J Med Vet Mycol 31:259, 1993.

Kaufman, L, et al: Comparative evaluation of commercial Premier EIA and microimmunodiffiusion and complement fixation tests for *Coccidioides immitis* antibodies. J Clin Microbiol 33:618, 1995.

Kaufman, L, et al: Immunodiffusion test for serodiagnosing subcutaneous zygomycosis. J Clin Microbiol 28:1887, 1990.

Kerr, JR: Suppression of fungal growth exhibited by *Pseudomonas aeruginosa*. J Clin Microbiol 32:525, 1994.

Kiska, DL, et al: Evaluation of new monoclonal antibody-based latex agglutination test for detection of cryptococcal polysaccharide antigen in serum and cerebrospinal fluid. *J Clin Microbiol* 32:2309, 1994.

Kwon-Chung, KJ and Bennett, J: Medical Mycology, Lea & Febiger, Philadelphia, 1992.

Laroche, R, et al: Cryptococcal meningitis association with acquired immunodeficiency syndrome in African patients: treatment with fluconazole. J Med Vet Mycol 30:71, 1992.

Lemieux, C, et al: Collaborative evaluation of antigen detection by a commercial latex agglutination test and ELISA in the diagnosis of invasive candidiasis. J Clin Microbiol 28:249, 1990.

Martins, TB, et al: Comparison of commercially available enzyme immunoassay with traditional serological tests for detection of antibodies to *Coccidioides immitis*. J Clin Microbiol 33:940, 1995.

McGinnis MR: Laboratory Handbook of Medical Mycology. Academic Press, New York, 1980.

Melcher, G, et al: Demonstration of a cell wall antigen cross-reacting with cryptococcal polysaccharide in experimental disseminated trichosporonosis. J Clin Microbiol 29:192, 1991.

Melchers, WJG, et al: General primer-mediated PCR for detection of *Aspergillus* species. J Clin Microbiol 32:1710, 1994.

Mikami, Y, et al: Synergistic postantifungal effect of flucytosine and fluconazole on *Candida albicans.* J Med Vet Mycol 30:197, 1992.

Millon, L, et al: Fluconazole-resistant recurrent oral candidiasis in human immunodeficiency virus-positive patients: persistence of *Candida albicans* strains with the same genotype. J Clin Microbiol 32:1115, 1994.

Miyakawa, Y, et al: New method for detection of *Candida albicans* in human blood by polymerase chain reaction. J Clin Microbiol 31:3344, 1993.

Nakamura, A, et al: Diagnosis of invasive candidiasis by detection of mannan antigen by using the avidin-biotin enzyme immunoassay. J Clin Microbiol 29:2363, 1991.

Nolte, FS: Use of selective buffered charcoal-yeast extract medium for isolation of nocardiae from mixed cultures. J Clin Microbiol 31:2554, 993.

Odds, FC: Long-term laboratory preservation of pathogenic yeasts in water. J Med Vet Mycol 29:413, 1991.

Padhye, AA, et al: Comparative evaluation of chemiluminescent DNA probe assays and exoantigen tests for rapid identification of *Blastomyces dermatitidis* and *Coccidioides immitis.* J Clin Microbiol 32:867, 1994.

Pfaller, MA, et al: Variations in fluconazole susceptibility and electrophoretic karyotype among oral isolates of *Candida albicans* from patients with AIDS and oral candidiasis. J Clin Microbiol 32:59, 1994.

Reboli, AC: Diagnosis of invasive candidiasis by dot immunobinding assay for *Candida* antigen detection. J Clin Microbiol 31:518, 1993.

Richardson, M and Warnock, D: Fungal Infection, Diagnosis and Management. Blackwell Scientific, Oxford, 1993.

Rodriguez-Tudela, JL and Aviles, P: Improved adhesive method for microscopic exam of fungi in culture. J Clin Microbiol 29:2604, 1991.

Ruhnke, M, et al: Emergence of fluconazole-resistant strains of *Candida albicans* in patients with recurrent oropharyngeal candidiosis and human immunodeficiency virus infection. J Clin Microbiol 32:2092, 1994.

Spreadbury, C, et al: Detection of *Aspergillus fumigatus* by polymerase chain reaction. J Clin Microbiol 31:615, 1993.

Standard, PG, et al: Exoantigen test for the rapid identification of *Exophiala spinifera.* J Med Vet Mycol 29:273, 1991.

Stockman, L, et al: Evaluation of commercially available acridinium ester-labelled chemiluminescent DNA probes for culture identification of *Blastomyces dermatitidis, Coccidioides immitis, Cryptococcus neoformans,* and *Histoplasma capsulatum.* J Clin Microbiol 31:845, 1993.

Tanner, DC, et al: Comparison of commercial kits for detection of cryptococcal antigen. J Clin Microbiol 32:1680, 1994.

Walsh, T, et al: *Trichosporon beigelii,* an emerging pathogen resistant to amphotericin B. J Clin Microbiol 28:1616, 1990.

Whittier, S, et al: Elimination of false-positive serum reactivity in latex agglutination test for cryptococcal antigen in human immunodeficiency virus-infected population. J Clin Microbiol 32:2158, 1994.

Zimmerman, S, et al: Evaluation of an enzyme-linked immunosorbent assay that uses ferous metal beads for determination of antihistoplasmal immunoglobulins G and M. J Clin Microbiol 28:59, 1990.

INTRODUCTION

Fungal culture and isolation is a boundless subject area. Almost every month, someone publishes a new fungal medium or procedure. Therefore, only the most widely accepted and used media, stains, and procedures will be discussed.

This module will progress in the same order of events as occurs in the clinical situation.

OBTAINING AND PROCESSING THE SPECIMEN

GENERAL CONSIDERATIONS

There are several general rules for good fungal specimen collection.

1. **Make sure the specimen is collected from the area most likely to be affected.** For example, when a hair infection is suspected, choose hair specimens that look broken and scaly, since these will be the ones most likely to contain organisms. For a sputum specimen, instruct the patient to produce material from a deep cough, not just spit up saliva.

2. **Use sterile technique in collecting the specimen.** Any fungus in the specimen may contaminate your hands and possibly cause an infection. Use only flamed and cooled forceps, sterile swabs, and specimen containers.

3. **The specimen must be adequate.** Often the physician will send down one swab to be used on bacteriology, tuberculosis, and fungal media. By the time the swab

is rolled over multiple media, any organisms present might be removed and the fungal culture could be falsely negative. If several cultures are requested, ask for additional swab specimens for use in mycology.

4. **The specimen must be promptly delivered to the laboratory and the laboratory must quickly process the specimen.** Slow-growing, **pathogenic** (disease-producing) fungi are rapidly overgrown by bacteria and fungal opportunists. If the specimen must sit before processing, refrigerate it. Besides keeping fungi alive and bacterial/fungal opportunist colony counts down, refrigeration prevents yeasts like *Candida albicans* from multiplying and therefore increasing their significance in the specimen. If the specimen must be mailed, add 50,000 units of penicillin and 100,000 μg of streptomycin, or alternatively, add 0.2 mg of chloramphenicol to each milliliter of material.

5. **The specimen must be adequately labelled, including the possible disease the physician suspects.** For certain fungal diseases, a special protocol is followed. For example, if actinomycosis is suspected, the specimen must be maintained, processed, and cultured under anaerobic conditions, or the causative (**etiologic**) organism will die. It must be remembered that the final laboratory results are only as good as the specimen that the laboratory has to work with.

SPECIFIC FUNGAL SPECIMEN SOURCES

See Chart 2–2 for fungal organisms that may be found in various specimens.

Blood and Bone Marrow

Commercial blood culture systems are now the norm, with fierce competition between the manufacturing companies for prominence in the marketplace. Many automated systems have gained acceptance. The ESP blood culture system (Difco) monitors cultures every 12 to 24 minutes by measuring headspace gas pressure. The BacT/Alert (Organon Teknika) and the BACTEC 9000 system (Becton-Dickinson Diagnostic Instrument Systems) both measure carbon dioxide production every 10 minutes. The older BACTEC NR system measures carbon dioxide twice a day for 2 days, then once a day thereafter. All these systems contain aerobic and anaerobic blood culture bottles, which support growth of bacteria and yeasts. BACTEC has an additional Fungal Medium, which enhances recovery of yeasts that might be overgrown by bacteria in mixed cultures.

Nonautomated commercial systems include Septi-Chek (Becton-Dickinson) and Isolator (Wampole Labs). Septi-Chek is a biphasic system in which inoculated broth is periodically inverted over three agars. The bottle should be vented and agitated constantly for the first 24 to 48 hours to improve yield. Isolator is a centrifugation-lysis system in which blood is collected into a special tube, the blood is lysed, the tube is centrifuged, and the pellet is inoculated to fungal agar media.

The blood specimen may be drawn into a transport Vacutainer tube with 0.35% polyantholsulfonate (SPS) for subsequent transfer into blood culture media once in the laboratory, or, alternatively, blood may be drawn directly into the blood culture media at the patient's bedside. The Isolator tube is drawn in a similar manner to the Vacutainer SPS tube. Most blood culture media contain SPS, which "inhibits complement and lysozyme activity, interferes with phagocytosis, and inactivates clinically achievable concentrations of aminoglycosides," according to Cumitech 1A, Blood Cultures II. If a nonautomated system is used (i.e., one that does not rely on carbon dioxide or gas pressure), 1 mL of 3% hydrogen peroxide can be added to each 50 mL of blood culture broth medium (not Isolator). The released catalase from breakdown of blood by hydrogen peroxide enhances yeast growth.

The most common fungal organism isolated from blood culture is *Candida* spp. Blood cultures are typically held for 7 days when bacterial pathogens are suspected, but they should be held for 3 weeks if a slow-growing fungal organism is suspected. All the blood culture systems adequately isolate yeasts, but only Isolator repeatedly isolates *H. capsulatum*, and none of the systems adequately isolates other filamentous fungi.

Bone marrow biopsy and culture can be useful in the diagnosis of histoplasmosis because blood may give a sparse yield. Other fungal organisms are better isolated from sites different than bone marrow. Because marrow is normally a sterile site, it can be inoculated to media without antibiotics. *Histoplasma* can be fastidious, thus nutrient-fortified media should be used. Hold cultures for 3 weeks before discarding as negative.

Cerebrospinal Fluid

Cerebrospinal fluid is aseptically collected as for bacteriology. The specimen is centrifuged, one drop of sediment is placed on a slide, a coverslip is added, and the mount is microscopically examined for fungal elements. More sediment direct mounts, particularly the India ink preparation and Wright stain, may be indicated, depending on the suspected agent. The remaining sediment is inoculated to aerobic fungal media (also include anaerobic media if *Actinomyces* is suspected).

Cutaneous: Hair, Nails, and Skin

Hair is plucked out by the roots with sterile forceps. Many fungi that infect hair will fluoresce with a Wood's lamp (366 nm). Hairs that fluoresce should be chosen for the specimen. If none of the hairs fluoresce, choose ones that are broken and scaly. Place the specimen in a sterile Petri dish for processing.

Nails are cleaned with 70% alcohol. With a sterile blade, scrape away and then dispose of the outer layers of nail. Scrape bits of the inner infected nail into a sterile Petri dish.

Skin is first cleaned with 70% alcohol to remove surface bacteria and fungal opportunists. If dermatophytosis is present, scrape the outer portions of the red ring with a sterile blade. If there is no ring, scrape areas that look most infected. Place the scrapings in a sterile Petri dish for processing.

In the laboratory, large skin and nail scrapings are cut into tiny sections. A small portion of soft skin or hair is mixed with potassium hydroxide, a coverslip is added, and the slide is gently warmed to aid clearing of tissue. The mount is examined microscopically for fungal elements. The rest of the specimen is inoculated onto fungal media.

If *Malassezia furfur* is a consideration, set up a SABHI tube layered with olive oil.

Respiratory: Bronchial Washings, Sputa, Throats, Transtracheal Aspirates

Usually the respiratory tract becomes infected with inhaled organisms. Many mycoses exhibit a pulmonary origin and then spread to other parts of the body.

Bronchial washings are obtained by threading a tube down the patient's throat to his bronchi, injecting a little sterile saline to pick up organisms in the lungs, and aspirating up the material. Since the tube passes down the throat, bronchial washings are usually contaminated with throat flora.

Sputa and bronchial washings should be collected upon rising in the morning. Overnight incubation and multiplication of fungi in the lungs will increase the chance of isolating fungi on culture. A 24-hour collection is discouraged because it becomes easily overgrown with bacterial and fungal contaminants. The patient should not eat before donating the specimen, as food left in the mouth may contain fungi that will grow on the patient's culture. The patient should brush his/her teeth, rinse with water, then produce material from a deep cough. This specimen is put in a sterile container and sent immediately to the laboratory. Since sputum is coughed up through the throat, it will be contaminated with normal oral flora.

Throat specimens are obtained by rolling two sterile swabs individually over the affected area. This should be performed prior to eating. The swabs are kept moist with 0.5 mL sterile saline until they are processed in the laboratory. If culturing for *Candida,* the organisms will not stick well to the swab. Therefore, scrape off material with a sterile tongue depressor, put the depressor in a sterile tube, and send it immediately to the laboratory.

Transtracheal aspirates are obtained by inserting a tube, through a surgically made slit in the trachea, down to the bronchi, and aspirating lung secretions. This procedure should be performed in the morning, when lung secretions have accumulated. Since this technique bypasses the throat, no throat flora contamination should be seen.

If actinomycosis is suspected, bronchial washings or transtracheal aspirates are sent to the laboratory as soon as possible for processing and anaerobic culturing, with explicit instructions to culture for *Actinomyces*. Respiratory swab specimens are immediately placed in an anaerobic transport container. If a syringe is used to obtain the specimen, be sure to seal the needle with a cork; utilize safety precautions when corking the needle.

Once in the laboratory, bronchial washings, sputa, and transtracheal aspirates are directly examined for blood, pus, or necrotic material, and these are plated.

If the specimen is tenacious or also to be used for TB culture, it is treated with an equal quantity of plain N-acetyl-L-cysteine (NALC) solution and vortexed to liquefy the mucus and equally distribute the organisms. Do not use specimens that have been treated with sodium hydroxide, which is routinely used for processing sputa for mycobacteria, as this chemical destroys many fungi. The NALC treated specimen is poured into a sterile 50 mL centrifuge tube, brought up to the 50 mL mark with 0.07 M phosphate buffer (pH 6.8–7.1), and mixed. If the specimen is to be used for TB culture, divide it into two tubes. Centrifuge both tubes at 2100 rpm for 15 minutes, and decant the supernatants. Place some of the sediment from the mycology tube onto appropriate media.

For the mycobacteriology tube, add 2 mL of 1.0% NaOH to the sediment, incubate 15 minutes, bring the volume up to the 50 mL mark with buffer, centrifuge as before, decant the supernatant, and inoculate the sediment to appropriate media.

A drop of concentrated sediment for fungus is put on a slide, a coverslip is added, and the specimen is examined under the microscope for budding yeasts, hyphae, spherules, or funguslike bacteria (Chart 2–1). Also various stains can be used as described in the section on direct examination of the specimen.

For the two throat swabs, roll one across a slide, stain, and examine for fungal elements. Roll the other swab across appropriate fungal media.

Tissue, Biopsies These specimens are obtained by the physician and should include both normal tissue and the center and edge of the lesion. They are kept moist with sterile saline until ready for processing. Tissues are aseptically teased apart in a sterile Petri dish and examined for granules and areas of pus or necrosis. Use these for culture. If granules are present, proceed as described under wounds, subcutaneous lesions, and mucocutaneous lesions. If areas of pus or necrosis are evident, inoculate these directly onto appropriate aerobic and anaerobic fungal media, smearing some on slides for a potassium hydroxide preparation and stained preparations. If there are no granules or areas of pus or necrosis, mince the rest of the tissue with a sterile scalpel and grind it in a tissue homogenizer. Inoculate the homogenized material onto the same media mentioned above and make direct smears. As with other specimens, if *Actinomyces* is suspected, the specimen must be processed under anaerobic conditions.

Urine Urine should be collected after overnight incubation in the bladder. Prostatic massage before urination may pick up *C. neoformans, B. dermatitidis, H. capsulatum,* or *C. immitis* causes of prostatitis, especially in acquired immunodeficiency syndrome (AIDS) patients. A clean catch or catheterized specimen is best, as this minimizes the presence of superficial genital flora. Twenty-four-hour urine specimens are discouraged because of overgrowth with opportunists. Urine should not be collected from a bedpan, as the pan may also contain opportunists. The urine specimen is placed in a sterile container and sent immediately to the laboratory.

In the laboratory, some of the urine is centrifuged and a direct mount for fungal exam is made with one drop of the sediment.

Stains may also be performed as indicated. If fungi are observed, a preliminary report is sent to the physician.

Usually urine is inoculated for bacteriology (calibrated loop, uncentrifuged urine, blood agar plate) and if fungi grow, they are quantitated and identified. Lately, the efficacy of quantitating fungi has been questioned. Classically, for a clean catch urine, over 100,000 fungal colonies of one kind per milliliter of urine were significant of infection; 10,000 to 100,000 were suspect; and under 10,000 or three different fungal/bacterial organisms present on the culture were representative of probable genital contamination. Now significance is based more on clinical findings, and identification is at the discretion of the individual physician. With urine obtained from a suprapubic puncture, any fungal colonies are significant and should be identified.

If an uncommon organism is suspected, the chance of recovery is increased if the urine is centrifuged and the sediment inoculated to fungal media. This procedure cannot be used to quantitate organisms; any fungi that grow are identified.

Vaginal, Uterine Cervix

These sites normally may contain yeasts. Usually the specimen is obtained to determine if these yeast flora, in particular *Candida albicans,* have overgrown their normal quantities to produce an infection. The specimen is collected with two sterile swabs, the swabs put in transport media,* for example, Stuart's or Amie's, and refrigerated until they are processed in the laboratory. Refrigeration slows multiplication of yeasts and bacterial normal flora.

In the laboratory, one swab is used to make a smear and stained for fungal elements. The other swab is rolled over fungal media. Any fungi that grow are semiquantitated (many, moderate, few) and identified.

Wounds, Subcutaneous Lesions, Mucocutaneous Lesions

In a wound, for example, a burn, the damaged tissue is very susceptible to infection and becomes easily colonized with fungal opportunists and yeasts. Also deep, ulcerated, and crusted subcutaneous and mucocutaneous lesions may be elicited by some fungi. Scrapings of the crusted portions and from the deep center and edge of active lesions are taken with a sterile scalpel. Remove the scrapings to 1 mL of sterile saline for transport. In addition to scrapings, material may be aspirated by needle and syringe from deep cysts or abscesses in the tissue. If there are any variously colored granules or tiny black dots, these are collected by laying sterile saline-wetted gauze on top of the lesion and pulling off the gauze. The granules should be trapped in the gauze mesh.

All specimens are kept in anaerobic containers in case *Actinomyces* is the causative agent. In the laboratory, a potassium hydroxide preparation is made with some of the scrapings or aspirate, and the mount is searched for fungal elements. The color of the granules is noted, since this may provide a clue as to the causative organism. Some of the granules are gently teased apart in a drop of sterile water or stained. They are observed microscopically for bacteria, funguslike bacteria, or hyphae interspersed with swollen chlamydosporelike cells. Some granules may contain a cementlike matrix or center of necrotic debris.

A potassium hydroxide preparation is made with some of the black dots; they are observed for thick-walled, dark-brown bodies (**sclerotic bodies**), which may be divided into two or four cells.

Concurrent with the direct mounts, the rest of the skin scrapings, aspirated material or black dots are inoculated to aerobic and anaerobic fungal media. The granules are washed several times in sterile saline to remove most contamination before culturing, then crushed and placed on media. Be sure to first plate the anaerobic agar and immediately place it under anaerobic conditions to ensure culture integrity.

STUDY QUESTIONS

1. List three general rules for good collection of fungal specimens.

2. Circle true or false:
   T   F   With a sputum culture, one would expect to observe growth of throat organisms.

3. Why is a urine specimen obtained upon rising in the morning?

---

*With the exception of *Candida albicans,* which survives well in most transport media, few data are available on the survival of other fungi. If an organism other than *C. albicans* is suspected, insert the swab into Sabouraud broth for transport.

4. Circle the letter of the correct answer:
   The fungal organism most commonly found in vaginal infections is:
   A. *Cryptococcus neoformans*

   B. *Coccidioides immitis*

   C. *Torulopsis glabrata*

   D. *Candida albicans*

   E. *Geotrichum candidum*

5. Circle true or false:
   T   F   Do not disinfect skin or nail areas with alcohol before taking scrapings, as the disinfectant will kill any pathogenic fungi you want to recover.

6. Circle true or false:
   T   F   Typically fungal infection is so overwhelming by the time it is isolated from blood or cerebrospinal fluid, there is no need to concentrate the specimen.

7. Circle true or false:
   T   F   Sputum specimens may be placed in plain N-acetyl-L-cysteine solution for concurrent fungal and TB processing.

8. Circle true or false:
   T   F   Granules from subcutaneous lesions only represent necrotic material and therefore should be disregarded.

STOP HERE UNTIL YOU HAVE COMPLETED THE ANSWERS.
Look up the answers in the back of the book. If you missed more than two, go back and review the sections on general considerations and specific sources of fungal specimens. Correctly complete any missed questions before proceeding further.

DIRECT EXAMINATION OF THE SPECIMEN

It is most important that each specimen be examined microscopically before, or concurrently with, culturing. A direct examination allows you to send out an immediate preliminary report to the physician.

With a positive direct examination result, you may also inoculate special media to quickly isolate and specifically identify the organism.

In the patient with an acute disease, direct examination results can possibly save his/her life. If a fungus is observed, the physician can immediately begin treatment. Some pathogenic fungi require a long incubation period (3 to 4 weeks) for growth. By this time the patient may have died, and isolation and identification of the causative fungal agent becomes academic.

On the other hand, if a fungus is not observed on a direct mount, the physician can avoid using antifungal drugs, which are generally toxic and require a long period of treatment. Also, the physician may start thinking about other possible disease agents.

It is obvious that to be of any use to the physician and patient you must be very careful and very thorough with the direct examination. Many times this may require performing more than one type of direct mount. Each type will now be discussed separately.

SALINE WET MOUNT

See box. Fungal elements that may be observed are budding yeasts, hyphae and pseudohyphae, conidia, thin branching filaments resembling bacteria (funguslike bacteria), granules, or *Coccidioides immitis* spherules. Chart 2–1 summarizes wet preparation findings.

SALINE WET MOUNT

Reagent Preparation
Saline:

Sodium chloride	0.85 g
Distilled water	100 mL

   1. Dissolve the sodium chloride in water and mix well.

Procedure
1. Place one drop of specimen on a glass slide and add one drop of saline.
2. Put on a coverslip and observe under low and high power under the microscope, using low light. Organisms will appear refractile, or shiny, and slightly green. Be sure to differentiate any yeast cells from bubbles or red blood cells: yeasts will contain inclusions, while the others will not.

LACTOPHENOL COTTON BLUE (LPCB) WET MOUNT
(Fig. 2–1)

See box. The phenol in the stain will kill any organisms, while the lactic acid preserves fungal structures. Cotton blue stains the chitin in fungal cell walls. The same structures may be seen as with the saline wet mount; however, the LPCB preparation can be made permanent.

LACTOPHENOL COTTON BLUE (LPCB) WET MOUNT

Reagent Preparation
LPCB: commercially available (Marion Scientific)

Phenol, concentrated	20 mL
Lactic acid	20 mL
Glycerol	40 mL
Cotton blue (China blue) (National Aniline Division)*	0.05 g
Distilled water	20 mL

   1. Dissolve cotton blue in distilled water, then add the rest of the ingredients. Mix well.

Procedure
1. Place one drop of specimen on a slide, and add one drop of LPCB. Some specimens, for example, pleural fluid, will precipitate with this stain.
2. Mix well and add a coverslip. Observe under the microscope for fungal elements; see Chart 2–1.
3. For a permanent preparation, rim the coverslip with clear nail polish or Permount.

*Cotton blue is a carcinogen, so handle with care. Trypan blue or aniline blue may be used instead. Lactophenol aniline blue is commercially available from Remel.

Text continues on page 44

CHART 2-1. STRUCTURES AND ASSOCIATED ORGANISMS COMMONLY SEEN IN SPECIMEN DIRECT EXAMINATIONS*

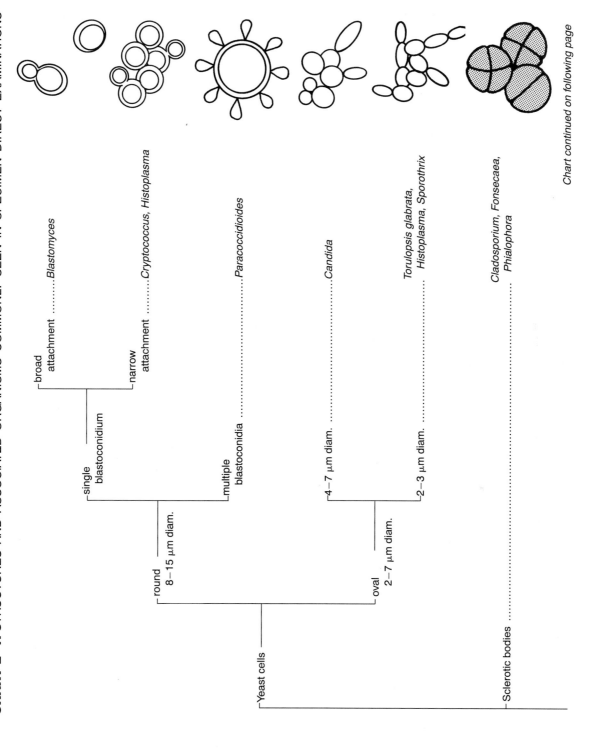

Yeast cells
- round 8—15 μm diam.
  - single blastoconidium
    - broad attachment .... *Blastomyces*
    - narrow attachment .... *Cryptococcus, Histoplasma*
  - multiple blastoconidia .... *Paracoccidioides*
- oval 2—7 μm diam.
  - 4—7 μm diam. .... *Candida*
  - 2—3 μm diam. .... *Torulopsis glabrata, Histoplasma, Sporothrix*

Sclerotic bodies .... *Cladosporium, Fonsecaea, Phialophora*

Chart continued on following page

CHART 2–1. STRUCTURES AND ASSOCIATED ORGANISMS COMMONLY SEEN IN SPECIMEN DIRECT EXAMINATIONS* (Continued)

Specimens other than hair, nail, and skin

Spherules
- 100–200 μm diam. .... *Rhinosporidium* 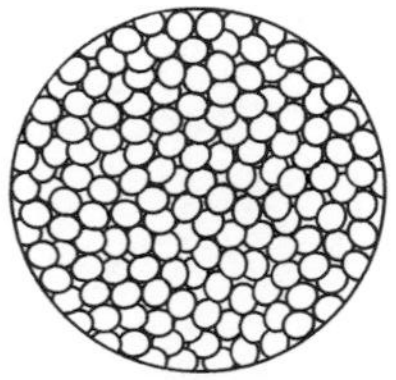
- 30–60 μm diam. .... *Coccidioides*

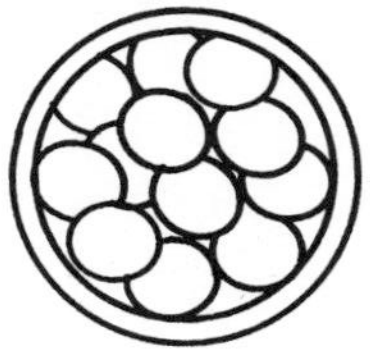

Granules
- round cells, darkly pigmented .... *Exophiala* 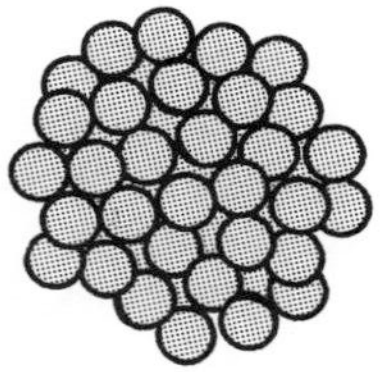
- cocci, 1 μm diam. .... Bacteria 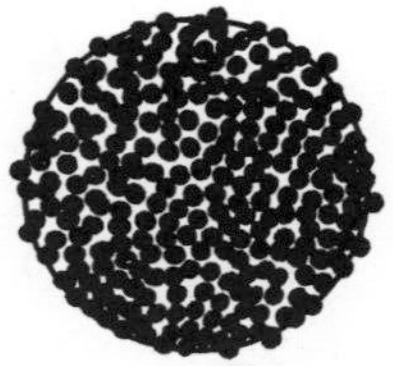
- filaments
  - 0.5–1 μm diam. .... Actinomycetes 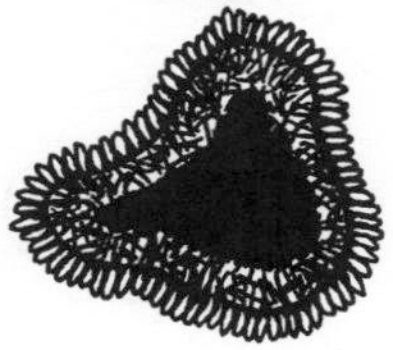
  - 3–4 μm diam. swollen cells common .... *Acremonium, Madurella, Scedosporium*

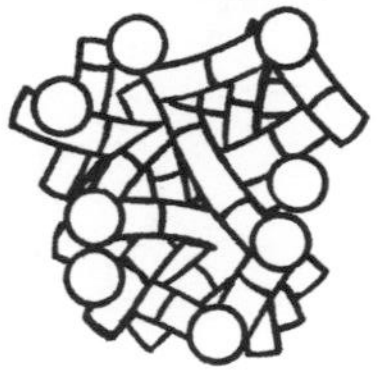

Chart continued on following page

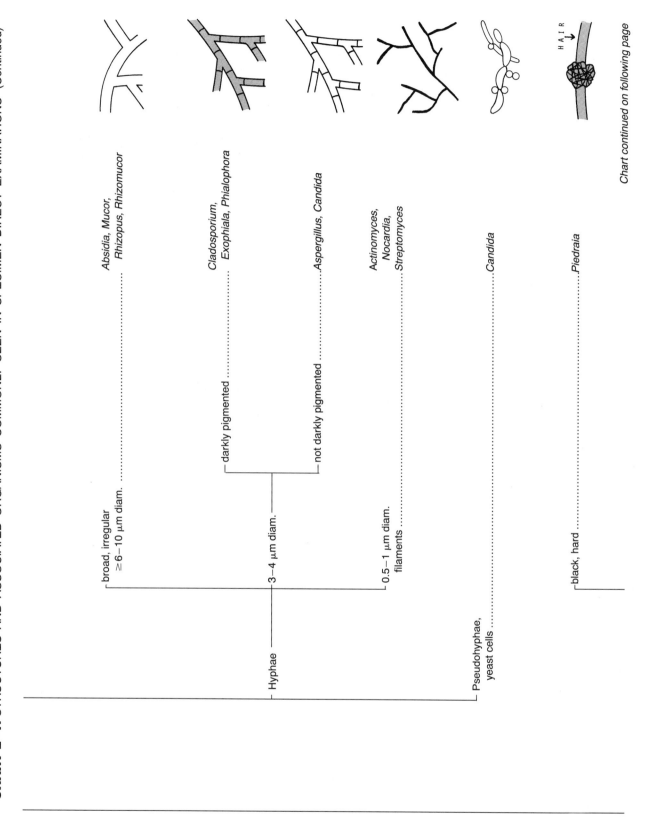

CHART 2-1. STRUCTURES AND ASSOCIATED ORGANISMS COMMONLY SEEN IN SPECIMEN DIRECT EXAMINATIONS* (Continued)

Hyphae ┬ broad, irregular ≥ 6 – 10 μm diam. .... *Absidia, Mucor, Rhizopus, Rhizomucor*

└ 3 – 4 μm diam. ┬ darkly pigmented .... *Cladosporium, Exophiala, Phialophora*

└ not darkly pigmented .... *Aspergillus, Candida*

0.5 – 1 μm diam. filaments .... *Actinomyces, Nocardia, Streptomyces*

Pseudohyphae, yeast cells .... *Candida*

black, hard .... *Piedraia*

Chart continued on following page

examination by wet prep or stained smears

hair
- nodules present
  - white, soft .... *Trichosporon*

- nodules absent, arthroconidia present
  - ectothrix .... *Microsporum, Trichophyton*

  - endothrix .... *Trichophyton*

nail
- hyphae
  - darkly pigmented .... *Hendersonula*

  - not darkly pigmented .... *Aspergillus, Epidermophyton, Microsporum, Scopulariopsis, Trichophyton*

Chart continued on following page

CHART 2-1. STRUCTURES AND ASSOCIATED ORGANISMS COMMONLY SEEN IN SPECIMEN DIRECT EXAMINATIONS* (Continued)

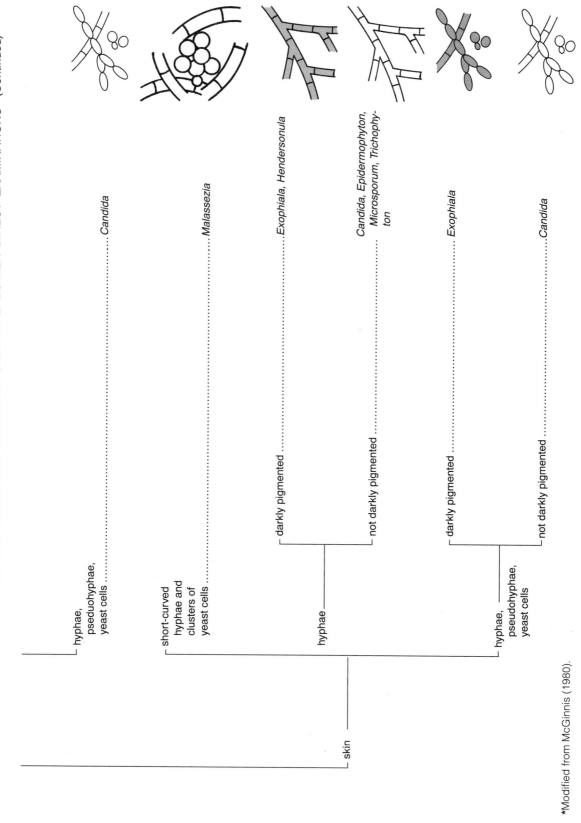

hyphae, pseduohyphae, yeast cells ...... *Candida*

short-curved hyphae and clusters of yeast cells ...... *Malassezia*

hyphae — darkly pigmented ...... *Exophiala, Hendersonula*

not darkly pigmented ...... *Candida, Epidermophyton, Microsporum, Trichophyton*

hyphae, pseudohyphae, yeast cells — darkly pigmented ...... *Exophiala*

not darkly pigmented ...... *Candida*

skin

*Modified from McGinnis (1980).

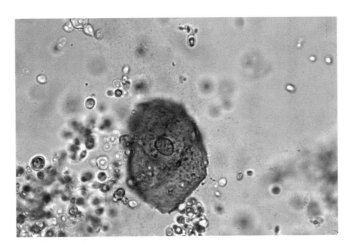

Figure 2–1. Lactophenol cotton blue (LPCB) wet mount, yeasts, and epithelial cell (magnification ×450).

POTASSIUM HYDROXIDE (KOH) PREPARATION
(Fig. 2–2)

If the specimen is skin, hair, or nail, the background cellular material may mask fungal elements. Potassium hydroxide will dissolve the keratin in these specimens, thus making any fungi more visible (see box). If there is a lot of cellular material in sputum or vaginal secretions, a KOH mount may be prepared to dissolve the background, thus making any yeasts more visible. However, a saline mount must be additionally done to quantitate epithelial cells and white blood cells and to note presence of *Trichomonas.*

POTASSIUM HYDROXIDE (KOH) PREPARATION

Reagent Preparation
10% potassium hydroxide: commercially available (Marion Scientific)

Potassium hydroxide	10 g
Glycerol	20 mL
Distilled water	80 mL

1. Dissolve the potassium hydroxide in water, then add glycerol. Glycerol prevents crystallization of the reagent and allows KOH preparations to be maintained for two days before drying up.

Procedure
1. Thinly smear some of the specimen on a glass slide.
2. Add one drop of 10% KOH, put on a coverslip, and gently heat by passing through a flame two or three times. Do not boil.
3. When the specimen has cleared (about 20 minutes), observe it under low and high power for any mycologic elements: hyphae, arthroconidia, and yeasts. On hair specimens, determine if the fungus is growing outside the hair shaft (**ectothrix invasion**) or inside the hair shaft (**endothrix invasion**). As with saline preparations, the organisms are not stained and thus they appear refractile. Low light is best for observing the fungi.

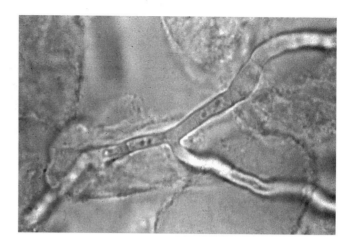

Figure 2–2. Potassium hydroxide (KOH) preparation, hyphae in scrapings. (Courtesy of Dr. Robert Kenney, William Beaumont Medical Center, El Paso, TX.)

GRAM STAIN
(Fig. 2–3)

Often, fungal presence is first noted on the routine specimen Gram stain performed for bacteriology. Fungi stain gram-positive, or blue. Any fungal forms may be observed, although yeasts and pseudohyphae are the most common.

Yeasts are two to three times larger than gram-positive cocci and will usually be budding if they are causing an infection. On a vaginal or urethral Gram-stained smear, a nonbudding yeast may be mistaken for a tailless spermatozoon. One must also be aware that on respiratory or CSF specimens, the capsule around *Cryptococcus neoformans* prevents definitive staining of the yeast itself, and thus the organism can easily be overlooked. This point is especially important since the physician may not order histologic stains or fungus cultures, and the patient's disease would remain undiagnosed. On a Gram stain, *C. neoformans* appears either as a round, pale lavender cell with gram-positive, granular inclusions, or as a gram-negative fat body.

Hyphae are two to three times wider than gram-positive rods, and often hyphae will not stain solidly inside, eliciting a granular appearance.

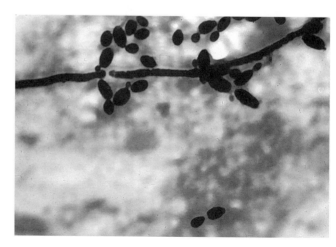

Figure 2–3. Gram stain, yeasts, and pseudohyphae (magnification ×1000).

ACID-FAST STAIN

The funguslike bacteria *Nocardia* are partially acid fast, appearing red against a blue background (see Color Plate 12), and may be mistaken for mycobacteria; however, *Nocardia* possess branching filaments as well as bacillary forms. The acid-fast stain for mycobacteria may overdecolorize *Nocardia*, giving false-negative results. Another smear should be made and stained with the modified Kinyoun acid-fast stain (see box) if *Nocardia* is suspected. These organisms may remain viable through the sputum digestion process for tuberculosis and will also grow on TB media. The disease caused by these funguslike bacteria may resemble tuberculosis; hence, the diagnosis of nocardiosis must always be considered when working up a patient for TB.

MODIFIED KINYOUN ACID-FAST STAIN

Reagent Preparation

Kinyoun's carbolfuchsin: commercially available (Difco)

Basic fuchsin	4 g
95% ethanol	20 mL
Phenol crystals	8 g
Distilled water	100 mL

1. Dissolve the basic fuchsin in ethanol.
2. Carefully add phenol and water. Mix well.

50% ethanol:

Concentrated (99–100%) ethyl alcohol	50 mL
Distilled water	50 mL

1. Mix the above ingredients together.

1% sulfuric acid:

Concentrated sulfuric acid	1 mL
Distilled water	99 mL

1. Carefully add acid to water and mix well.

Methylene blue: commercially available (Difco)

Methylene blue	2.5 g
95% ethanol	100 mL

1. Dissolve methylene blue in alcohol and mix well.

Procedure

1. Make smears of the organism* and positive and negative controls. Heat fix.
2. Flood the slides with Kinyoun's carbolfuchsin. Stain for 5 minutes.
3. Wash with tap water.
4. Flood the slides with 50% ethanol until all excess dye is removed. This step removes precipitated dye, eliminating a lot of background debris.
5. Wash with tap water.
6. Decolorize with 1% sulfuric acid for 3 minutes.†
7. Wash with tap water.
8. Counterstain with methylene blue for 1 minute.
9. Wash with tap water and allow the slides to air dry. *Nocardia* stains red, while other bacteria and fungi are blue. If this procedure is used for yeast ascospore production, asci stain red, while blastoconidia are blue.

---

*Nocardia should be taken from cultures on 7H10 or 7H11 agar, as these media enhance acid fastness.

†Acid alcohol for staining mycobacteria may be used for decolorization instead. Acid alcohol is flooded on the slides for 5 seconds and washed off. This method gives variable results and is thus not recommended.

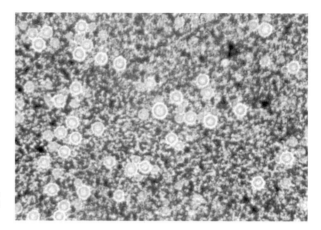

Figure 2–4. India ink preparation, *Cryptococcus neoformans* (magnification ×1000).

INDIA INK PREPARATION (Fig. 2–4)

This procedure is employed to observe capsules around yeasts, especially *Cryptococcus neoformans* in cerebrospinal fluid sediment (see box). Unfortunately, all bacterial and fungal organisms, encapsulated or not, will stand out distinctly against the black India ink background, because the ink will not penetrate the cell wall or capsule. Therefore, be careful to search for capsules only. Some bacteria, for example, *Klebsiella*, possess capsules that may be mistaken for yeasts. However, bacteria are one fourth the size of yeasts, and bacteria will not be budding. Some laboratories use a positive India ink preparation as definitive evidence for the presence of *Cryptococcus neoformans*. It must be emphasized that other *Cryptococcus* species, as well as *Rhodotorula, Torulopsis, Sporobolomyces, Trichosporon beigelii,* and *Prototheca stagnora* (an alga that may be confused with *Cryptococcus*) may be encapsulated. The laboratory must perform other studies, such as dark brown pigment production on caffeic acid agar, direct antigen testing, or specific carbohydrate assimilation reactions, before calling an organism *Cryptococcus neoformans*. See Module 5 for further information on *Cryptococcus*.

INDIA INK PREPARATION

Reagent Preparation
India ink or nigrosin

Procedure
1. On a slide, mix a *tiny* drop of India ink or nigrosin,*† with one drop of specimen sediment, add a coverslip, and let the mount sit 10 minutes to allow yeast cells to settle into one plane of focus.
2. Observe the preparation under the microscope, with the condenser adjusted for maximum light, for capsules around budding yeasts.

---

*Marion Scientific

†I prefer nigrosin over India ink because nigrosin provides a homogenized background, which facilitates the search for capsules.

CALCOFLUOR WHITE STAIN

Calcofluor white, a bleaching agent used in the paper and textile industry, is taken up into the chitin of the fungal cell wall; background human material does not possess chitin, thus the dye is not absorbed into human tissue. The dye in the fungus produces a chalk-white or apple-green fluorescence depending upon excitation wavelength (usually 340 nm) when observed under an ultraviolet microscope (Fig. 2–5). In a particularly hard specimen such as nail, calcofluor white may be mixed with 10% KOH just immediately before use to dissolve background material. Calcofluor will not fluoresce inside *Coccidioides* spherules, and vaginal wet preparations are difficult to interpret (Hageage and Harrington 1984).

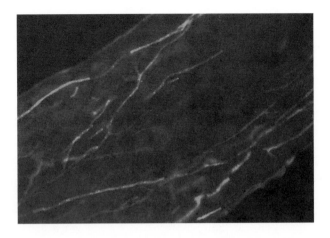

Figure 2–5. Calcofluor white fluorescent–stained fungus in hair. (From Hageage and Harrington, 1984, with permission.)

CALCOFLUOR WHITE—KOH PREPARATION

Reagent Preparation
Calcofluor white:

Calcofluor white *M2R* powder (Polysciences)	0.1 g
Distilled water	100 mL

1. Gently heat distilled water and dissolve calcofluor white.
2. Cool.

10% KOH (see page 44)

Procedure
1. Mix 1 drop calcofluor white and 1 drop 10% KOH on a microscope slide.
2. Mix the specimen with the solution, coverslip, and examine under the ultraviolet (UV) microscope for fungal elements, which fluoresce.

OTHER STAINS

Stains for fungal detection may be performed in laboratory sections other than microbiology. The technologists in histology perform the Gomori methenamine silver (GMS) stain, in which fungi and actinomycetes appear black against a green background (see Color Plate 13), and the periodic acid-Schiff (PAS) stain, in which fungal elements, but not actinomycetes, look magenta against a light pink or green background (see Color Plate 64). They can also perform Mayer's mucicarmine stain when *Cryptococcus* is suspected. The capsules of these organisms appear red against a yellow background, while other similar-appearing fungi do not take up the red stain. The hematoxylin and eosin (H&E) stain is the workhorse of pathologists: the background is pink, with tissue nuclei and fungal elements staining purple (see Color Plate 57). An added advantage to the H&E preparation is that stained sections may be placed directly under a fluorescent microscope (340 nm wavelength) where fungi such as *Blastomyces, Cryptococcus, Candida, Aspergillus, Coccidioides, Paracoccidioides,* and occasionally *Histoplasma* will brightly autofluoresce while tissue and background material remain dark.

The hematology technologists perform the Wright stain on blood and bone marrow smears to look for purple pseudoencapsulated yeast forms of *Histoplasma capsulatum* inside polymorphonuclear cells and monocytes.

The Fontana-Masson stain may be used to differentiate dematiaceous fungi from hyaline fungi in tissue. The melaninlike pigment in dematiaceous fungi stains positive, whereas hyaline fungi are negative (Friedman et al. 1991).

STUDY QUESTIONS

1. Why is it important to perform a direct mount examination on every specimen? Give two reasons.

Matching: Place the letter of the answer in Column B in front of the words in Column A.

Column A

2. _____ KOH preparation
3. _____ Acid-fast stain
4. _____ India ink preparation
5. _____ Wright stain
6. _____ Gram stain
7. _____ Calcofluor white preparation

Column B

A. *Nocardia*
B. *Histoplasma capsulatum*
C. Fungi stain magenta
D. Hair
E. Fungi fluoresce
F. *Cryptococcus neoformans*
G. Fungi stain blue

8. Circle true or false:
   T   F   With the India ink preparation, only encapsulated organisms are visible against the black background.

9. Circle the letter of the correct answer.
   Which is the most useful mounting fluid for nail scrapings?
   A. Lactophenol cotton blue
   B. Acetic acid
   C. Saline
   D. Potassium hydroxide

10. Circle true or false:
    T   F   With specimen lactophenol cotton blue mounts, which show fungi, the specimen may be removed from under the coverslip and cultured.

STOP HERE UNTIL YOU HAVE COMPLETED THE ANSWERS.
Look up the answers in the back of the book. If you missed more than one, go back and review the section on direct examinations. Correctly complete any missed questions before proceeding further.

CULTURING THE SPECIMEN

PRIMARY FUNGAL MEDIA

Concurrent with examining the direct mount, specific fungal media are inoculated to initially isolate any organisms (primary media). Tubed media are preferred over plates, as the former will not dry out over the long incubation period, and also this reduces the chance for fungal reproductive structures to become airborne and contaminate the room and people. Never use plates when *Coccidioides immitis* is suspected, as this fungus is extremely infectious and aerosols may be inhaled. Always work under a biological safety cabinet, wear gloves, autoclave specimens and inoculated media when finished, and disinfect the work area daily. See individual sections on specimen collection and processing, also Chart 2–2 for media to be inoculated for various specimens. Note that *Pseudomonas* in a specimen can inhibit growth of most *Candida, T. glabrata, S. cerevisiae,* and *A. fumigatus* from the same specimen (Kerr 1994).

The goal is to isolate all the possible pathogens. For this a combination of nonselective and selective media (i.e., with or without antibiotics) is necessary. Also, because some systemic fungal pathogens are fastidious, use media with blood for extra nutrition.

CHART 2–2. FUNGI THAT MAY BE ISOLATED FROM VARIOUS SPECIMENS AND SUGGESTED PRIMARY ISOLATION MEDIA

Specimen	Normal Fungal Flora	Potential Fungal Pathogens	Primary Isolation Media
Blood, bone marrow	None	Any growth of *Candida* sp. *Histoplasma capsulatum* *Cryptococcus neoformans* Other organisms that have become systemic *Blastomyces dermatitidis*	Brain heart infusion broth with blood or commercial blood culture medium
Cerebrospinal fluid	None	Any growth of *Coccidioides immitis* *Histoplasma capsulatum* *Actinomyces* *Nocardia* *Candida* sp. *Cryptococcus neoformans* Opportunists repeatedly isolated	Brain heart infusion agar with blood Anaerobic brain heart infusion agar with blood
Hair	Possibly a few opportunists	Common: Any growth of *Trichophyton* *Microsporum* Uncommon: Any growth of *Piedraia hortai* *Trichosporon beigelii*	Inhibitory mold agar Dermatophyte test medium
Mucocutaneous scrapings	None	Any growth of *Candida* sp. *Paracoccidioides brasiliensis* Microscopic observation of *Rhinosporidium seeberi*	Sabouraud brain heart infusion agar Inhibitory mold agar Brain heart infusion agar with blood, gentamicin, and chloramphenicol* Brain heart infusion agar with blood, gentamicin, chloramphenicol, cycloheximide*
Nail scrapings	None	Any growth of *Candida* sp. *Trichophyton* *Epidermophyton* *Aspergillus* *Scopulariopsis*	Inhibitory mold agar Dermatophyte test medium

Skin scrapings	Possibly a few contaminants
	Possibly a few yeast (*Candida*)
		Common:
		Moderate-heavy growth of *Candida* sp.
		Any growth of *Trichophyton*
		Microsporum
		Epidermophyton
		Uncommon:
		Any growth of opportunists repeatedly isolated
		    Cryptococcus
		    Malassezia furfur
		    Exophiala werneckii
		    Blastomyces dermatitidis
		    Paracoccidioides brasiliensis
		    Coccidioides immitis
		    Histoplasma capsulatum
		    Agents of chromoblastomycosis
		      (*Fonsecaea, Phialophora, Cladosporium*)
		    Agents of mycetoma
		      (*Scedosporium, Exophiala,*
		      (*Nocardia, Streptomyces,*
		      (*Actinomyces*)
			Inhibitory mold agar
			Dermatophyte test medium
			Sabouraud brain heart infusion agar layered with olive oil (if suspect *Malassezia*)
			Brain heart infusion agar with blood, gentamicin, chloramphenicol, cycloheximide*

Chart continued on following page

CHART 2–2. FUNGI THAT MAY BE ISOLATED FROM VARIOUS SPECIMENS AND SUGGESTED PRIMARY ISOLATION MEDIA (Continued)

Specimen	Normal Fungal Flora	Potential Fungal Pathogens	Primary Isolation Media
Sputum, bronchial washings	Few yeast (Candida) Few opportunists	Common: Moderate-heavy growth of Candida sp. (esp. C. albicans) or T. glabrata Moderate-heavy growth of opportunists repeatedly isolated (esp. Aspergillus, Rhizopus, Mucor, Penicillium, Geotrichum) Uncommon: Any growth of Nocardia Actinomyces Cryptococcus neoformans Blastomyces dermatitidis Paracoccidioides brasiliensis Coccidioides immitis Histoplasma capsulatum Sporothrix schenckii Moderate-heavy growth of Saccharomyces	Sabouraud brain heart infusion agar Inhibitory mold agar Brain heart infusion agar with blood, gentamicin, chloramphenicol Brain heart infusion agar with blood, gentamicin, chloramphenicol, cycloheximide Birdseed agar (AIDS patients) Nocardia medium if suspected
Subcutaneous lesions and abscesses	None	Any growth of Candida sp. Opportunists repeatedly isolated Agents of chromoblastomycosis (Fonsecaea, Phialophora, Cladosporium) Agents of mycetoma (Scedosporium, Exophiala, Nocardia, Streptomyces, Actinomyces) Sporothrix schenckii Coccidioides immitis Blastomyces dermatitidis Cryptococcus neoformans Histoplasma capsulatum Wangiella	Sabouraud brain heart infusion agar Inhibitory mold agar Brain heart infusion agar with blood, gentamicin, chloramphenicol Brain heart infusion agar with blood, gentamicin, chloramphenicol, cycloheximide
Throat	Few yeast (Candida) Few opportunists	Common: Moderate-heavy growth of Candida albicans Uncommon: Moderate-heavy growth of Geotrichum candidum Saccharomyces cerevisiae	Sabouraud brain heart infusion agar
Tissue, biopsy material	None	Any growth of Paracoccidioides brasiliensis (lymph nodes) Agents of zygomycosis (Rhizopus, Mucor, Absidia, Mortierella, Cunninghamella) repeatedly isolated Agents of mycetoma (Scedosporium, Nocardia, Streptomyces, Actinomyces) Microscopic observation of Rhinosporidium seeberi	Sabouraud brain heart infusion agar Inhibitory mold agar Brain heart infusion agar with blood, gentamicin, chloramphenicol Brain heart infusion agar with blood, gentamicin, chloramphenicol, cycloheximide Nocardia, medium if suspected
Transtracheal aspirate	None	Same as for sputum, bronchial washings	Same as for sputum, bronchial washings

Chart continued on following page

CHART 2–2. FUNGI THAT MAY BE ISOLATED FROM VARIOUS SPECIMENS AND SUGGESTED PRIMARY ISOLATION MEDIA (Continued)

Specimen	Normal Fungal Flora	Potential Fungal Pathogens	Primary Isolation Media
Urine	None from catheterized specimen	Common: Over 100,000 colonies/mL of *Candida* sp. (esp. *C. albicans*) or *T. glabrata* Uncommon: Any growth of *Blastomyces dermatitidis* *Coccidioides immitis* *Histoplasma capsulatum* *Cryptococcus neoformans*	Sabouraud brain heart infusion agar Inhibitory mold agar Brain heart infusion agar with blood, gentamicin, chloramphenicol* Brain heart, infusion agar with blood, gentamicin, chloramphenicol, cycloheximide* Birdseed agar (AIDS patients)
Vaginal, uterine, cervix	Few to moderate number of yeast colonies (*Candida*)	Common: Heavy growth of *Candida albicans* or *T. glabrata* Uncommon: Heavy growth of *Geotrichum candidum*	Sabouraud brain heart infusion agar Inhibitory mold agar
Wound	None	Any growth of *Candida* sp. Opportunistic pathogens repeatedly isolated	Sabouraud brain heart infusion agar Inhibitory mold agar Brain heart infusion agar with blood, gentamicin, chloramphenicol Brain heart infusion agar with blood, gentamicin, chloramphenicol, cycloheximide

*Inoculate this medium if *Histoplasma*, *Paracoccidioides*, or *Blastomyces* is suspected.

Nonselective Media

Sabouraud Brain Heart Infusion Agar (SABHI)

SABHI is becoming the medium of choice for general initial isolation, because the traditional Sabouraud dextrose agar (SDA) is not as rich nutritionally and thus will not support growth of as many fungi. SABHI allows bacteria, fungal opportunists, dermatophytes, yeasts, subcutaneous pathogens, and most systemic pathogens to grow. Some fastidious strains of *H. capsulatum* and *B. dermatitidis* may not prosper. SABHI is commercially available.

SABOURAUD BRAIN HEART INFUSION AGAR (SABHI)

Medium Preparation: commercially available (Difco, BBL)

Dextrose	40 g
Neopeptone (Difco)	10 g
Brain heart infusion	37 g
Agar	15 g
Distilled water	1 L

1. Mix together the above ingredients and heat to dissolve.
2. Tube in 15 mL aliquots and autoclave at 15 psi for 10 minutes. Slant so there is a 1-inch end, cool, and refrigerate.

Procedure

1. Bring the tube to room temperature. Swab the entire surface of the agar slant. Push specimen gently into the agar. If media with antibiotics are also to be inoculated, be sure to swab plain SABHI and brain heart infusion agar with blood first so there is no antibiotic carryover.
2. Incubate with the cap loose, at 30° C for 1 month before discarding as negative.

Brain Heart Infusion Agar with Blood (BHIB)

This general medium is nutritionally richer than SABHI and thus should be reserved for specimens from normally sterile sites or for anaerobic actinomycetes.

BRAIN HEART INFUSION AGAR WITH BLOOD (BHIB)

Medium Preparation: commercially available(Difco, Remel)

Brain heart infusion	37 g
Agar	20 g
Distilled water	1 L
Sheep blood, defibrinated, sterile	100 mL

1. Mix together the brain heart infusion, agar, and water. Autoclave at 15 psi for 15 minutes and cool to 50° C.
2. While swirling the flask, add the sheep blood, then immediately pour into plates or aseptically aliquot in tubes and slant. Cool completely and refrigerate. If medium is to be used for anaerobic actinomycetes, prereduce it in an anaerobic chamber before inoculating.

Procedure

1. Bring the medium to room temperature. If it is to be used for dimorphic mold conversion, follow instructions in Module 7.
2. If it is to be used for anaerobic actinomycetes, swab one third of the prereduced plate, then streak out for isolation. Granules from specimens are first washed several times with sterile saline, crushed, then smeared on one third of the agar plate, before streaking for isolation. Try to maintain anaerobic conditions from time of specimen collection through processing, to incubation. Set inoculated media in an anaerobic chamber at 37° C for 7 to 10 days before discarding as negative.

Sabouraud Dextrose Agar (SDA)

This general medium has an acid pH of 5.6 and is nutritionally poor (see box). These conditions inhibit growth of many bacteria but allow fungal opportunists and pathogenic fungi to grow, with the exception of *Histoplasma capsulatum* and some strains of *Nocardia asteroides*.

SABOURAUD DEXTROSE AGAR (SDA)

Medium Preparation: commercially available (Difco, BBL)

Dextrose	40 g
Neopeptone (Difco)	10 g
Agar	15 g
Distilled water	1 L

1. Mix together the above ingredients and heat to dissolve.
2. Tube in 15 mL aliquots and autoclave at 15 psi for 10 minutes. Slant so there is a 1-inch end, cool, and refrigerate.

Procedure

1. Bring the tube to room temperature. Swab the entire surface of the agar slant. Pieces of specimen are pushed slightly into the agar. If media with antibiotics are also to be inoculated, be sure to swab plain Sabouraud dextrose agar and brain heart infusion agar with blood first so there is no antibiotic carryover.
2. Incubate with the cap loose, at 30° C for 1 month before discarding as negative.

Selective Media with Antibiotics

Gentamicin, chloramphenicol, and cycloheximide are frequently added in different combinations to media to select for various fungi. Gentamicin inhibits bacteria, chloramphenicol inhibits funguslike bacteria and yeast phases of dimorphic fungi, and cycloheximide inhibits funguslike bacteria, many yeasts, and many fungal opportunists. (See Chart 2–3.)

Inhibitory Mold Agar (IMA)

This medium is commercially available (Remel, BBL). It contains gentamicin, which inhibits bacteria but allows growth of yeasts, fungal opportunists, and pathogenic fungi including dermatophytes and some *H. capsulatum.*

Brain Heart Infusion Agar with Blood, Gentamicin, and Chloramphenicol

This medium is commercially available (B3 agar, Remel). Blood makes it especially nutritious, and the gentamicin and chloramphenicol inhibit bacteria. *Nocardia* and other aerobic actinomycetes will not grow, but fungal opportunists and fastidious fungal pathogens (*H. capsulatum* and *B. dermatitidis*) grow well.

Brain Heart Infusion Agar with Blood, Gentamicin, Chloramphenicol, and Cycloheximide

This medium is commercially available (B4 agar, Remel). It is best used for fastidious fungal pathogens. Bacteria, aerobic actinomycetes, and fungal opportunists will be inhibited.

Dermatophyte Test Medium (DTM)

DTM is commercially available (Medical Technology Corp), and is frequently used in dermatology offices. It contains antibiotics plus a phenol red indicator; when dermatophytes grow, they change the color from yellow to red, although a few fungi other than dermatophytes can accomplish this also.

CHART 2–3. PATHOGENIC FUNGI INHIBITED BY CYCLOHEXIMIDE AND CHLORAMPHENICOL

Cycloheximide Inhibits:	Chloramphenicol Inhibits:
Scedosporium apiospermum	*Nocardia asteroides*†
Cryptococcus neoformans	*Nocardia brasiliensis*
Cryptococcus sp.	
Candida parapsilosis	Other funguslike bacteria
Candida krusei	Yeast phases of dimorphic fungi*
Candida tropicalis	
Candida rugosa	
Torulopsis glabrata	
Yeast phases of dimorphic fungi*	
Actinomyces sp.	
Nocardia sp.	
Streptomyces sp.	
Aspergillus fumigatus†	
Penicillium sp.	
Geotrichum sp.	
Scopulariopsis sp.	
Saccharomyces sp.	
Absidia sp.	
Mucor sp.	
Rhizopus sp.	

*Yeast phases are inhibited only at 37° C, not 25° C.
†Partially inhibited.

Special Considerations

If *Nocardia* is suspected, paraffin may be added to the nonselective fungal medium; it inhibits bacterial overgrowth and enhances growth of *Nocardia*. Also, *Nocardia* grows well on *7H11* mycobacterial medium. The *Legionella* nonselective buffered charcoal-yeast extract agar (BCYE agar) and other selective *Legionella* agars are useful as primary media for isolation of *Nocardia* from contaminated respiratory specimens such as sputum (Nolte, 1993).

Sputum from AIDS patients may be plated on birdseed agar (caffeic acid agar) to selectively isolate **Cryptococcus neoformans.** This medium prevents overgrowth of bacteria, and *C. neoformans* will grow dark brown while other yeasts will be white or beige. Birdseed agar is commercially available.

If **Actinomyces** is suspected, plate the specimen onto brain heart infusion agar with blood (no antibiotics) as soon as possible after collection, and immediately incubate under anaerobic conditions at 35–37° C.

INCUBATION TEMPERATURE

Fungal cultures should be generally incubated at 30° C. Room temperature (25° C) is acceptable, although some organisms may multiply slower at this temperature. A 37° C incubation may actually inhibit some fungi. Since so few dimorphic fungi are recovered, it is preferable first to isolate them in the mold phase (room temperature or 30° C), then set up cultures at 37° C for conversion to the yeast phase.

INCUBATION TIME

Some fungi mature within 3 to 4 days, while others may require 3 to 4 weeks. (See Chart 2–4 for incubation times of various organisms.) Growth rates may vary, depending on conditions such as media used, temperature of incubation, or inhibitors in the patient's specimen. To reduce the risk of false-negative reports, keep all cultures at least 1 month before reporting final results and discarding media. Incubate cultures suspected of containing *H. capsulatum* for 12 weeks before discarding as negative. Maintaining a moist atmosphere (40 to 50% humidity) helps keep inoculated media from drying out and enhances fungal growth. Seal plates with air-permeable tape to prevent contamination and keep screw caps loose.

SUBCULTURE MEDIA

Once fungi have grown on primary culture, they frequently need subculturing for complete isolation. In addition, subculture media are used to promote identification. Yeasts are subcultured to neutral Sabouraud dextrose agar (Emmon's modification), which is commercially available (Remel). This medium has less glucose and a neutral pH compared to regular Sabouraud dextrose agar, which allows for better maintenance of yeasts. Yeasts can also be subcultured to birdseed agar for quick identification of *Cryptococcus neoformans* (see Yeast chapter). Molds are transferred to potato dextrose agar, which promotes sporulation and pigmentation of colonies.

NEUTRAL SABOURAUD DEXTROSE AGAR (EMMON'S MODIFICATION)

Medium preparation: commercially available (Remel, Difco)

Glucose	20 g
Neopeptone	10 g
Agar	20 g
Distilled water	1 L

Procedure:
1. Dissolve ingredients into distilled water.
2. Sterilize in autoclave at 121° C for 15 minutes. Adjust pH to 6.8–7.0 and pour plates.

CHART 2–4. GROWTH RATES OF VARIOUS FUNGI

Growth Rate	Molds	Yeasts	Funguslike Bacteria
Rapid growers (form mature colonies in 5 days or less)	Fungal opportunists: Absidia, Acremonium, Alternaria, Aspergillus, Aureobasidium, Chrysosporium, Cladosporium, Curvularia, Bipolaris, Exserohilum, Fusarium, Mucor, Nigrospora, Paecilomyces, Penicillium, Rhizopus, Scopulariopsis, Sepedonium, Syncephalastrum, Trichoderma Subcutaneous: Dimorphic—Sporothrix schenckii	Candida Cryptococcus Geotrichum Rhodotorula Saccharomyces Torulopsis Trichosporon Subcutaneous: Dimorphic conversion— Sporothrix schenckii Systemic: Dimorphic conversion— Blastomyces dermatitidis	Actinomyces (anaerobic only) spider colonies at 5 days (rapid growth) classic molar tooth colonies at 8 days (intermediate growth) Nocardia Streptomyces Actinomadura Nocardiopsis
Intermediate growers (form mature colonies in 6 to 10 days)	Dermatophytes: Epidermophyton floccosum Microsporum canis, distortum, gypseum, nanum, vanbreuseghemii Trichophyton ajelloi, mentagrophytes Subcutaneous: Scedosporium apiospermum Systemic: Dimorphic—Coccidioides immitis	Systemic: Dimorphic conversion— Histoplasma capsulatum	
Slow growers (form mature colonies in 11 to 21 days)	Dermatophytes: Microsporum audouinii Trichophyton rubrum, schoenleinii, tonsurans, verrucosum, violaceum Subcutaneous: Cladosporium carrionii Exophiala jeanselmei Fonsecaea compacta, pedrosoi Phialophora verrucosa Systemic: Dimorphic—Blastomyces dermatitidis, Histoplasma capsulatum, Paracoccidioides brasiliensis	Systemic: Dimorphic (primary growth)— Paracoccidioides brasiliensis	

POTATO DEXTROSE AGAR (PDA)

Medium preparation: commercially available (Difco)

Potato flakes, for example,	
Betty Crocker Potato Buds	20 g
Glucose	10 g
Agar	15 g
Distilled water	1 L

Procedure:
1. Mix together the above ingredients and autoclave at 15 psi for 15 minutes.
2. While frequently swirling the flask, pour plates of medium 4 mm thick. Cool and refrigerate.

**STUDY
QUESTIONS**

Circle the correct answer for questions 1 to 4:

1. The best medium to isolate fungal opportunists from a nonsterile site is:
   A. Dermatophyte test medium
   B. Inhibitory mold agar
   C. Brain heart infusion agar with blood, gentamicin, chloramphenicol, and cycloheximide
   D. Brain heart infusion agar with blood

2. The best medium to isolate fastidious *Histoplasma capsulatum* from sputum is:
   A. Sabouraud brain heart infusion agar
   B. Brain heart infusion agar with blood
   C. Inhibitory mold agar
   D. Brain heart infusion agar with blood, gentamicin, chloramphenicol, and cycloheximide

3. The best medium to isolate yeasts from a vaginal specimen is:
   A. Brain heart infusion agar with blood, gentamicin, and chloramphenicol
   B. Brain heart infusion agar with blood, gentamicin, chloramphenicol, and cycloheximide
   C. Sabouraud brain heart infusion agar
   D. 7H10 agar

4. The best medium to isolate *Cryptococcus neoformans* in bronchial washings from an AIDS patient is:
   A. Sabouraud brain heart infusion agar
   B. Brain heart infusion agar with gentamicin, chloramphenicol, and cycloheximide
   C. Inhibitory mold agar
   D. Birdseed agar

5. According to this module, what is an intermediate growth rate?

6. Circle true or false.
   T   F   Potato dextrose agar promotes sporulation.

STOP HERE UNTIL YOU HAVE COMPLETED THE ANSWERS.
Look up the answers in the back of the book. If you missed more than two of them, go back and review the section on primary fungal media and incubation time and temperature. Correctly complete any missed questions before proceeding further.

**EXAMINING THE
CULTURE**

Once a mature colony has formed, observe it for macroscopic appearance. Module 1 contains descriptive terms of colonial morphology. Colonial appearance may help to identify a fungus. However, this morphology may vary greatly between fungal strains, times and temperatures of incubation, and culture media. For molds, the final identification is basically dependent on microscopic morphology, although there are a few useful biochemical tests. For yeasts and funguslike bacteria, biochemical tests are the primary basis for identification, with less emphasis on microscopic and macroscopic appearance. There are several frequently used procedures to microscopically examine a culture.

**TEASE MOUNT
METHOD**

See box and Figure 2–6. The advantage of this method is that it can be performed and examined immediately after maturation of the fungal colony on the primary isolation plate. The disadvantage is that the rough action of teasing apart hyphae disturbs the position of conidia so that oftentimes the structural morphology of the organism cannot be discerned.

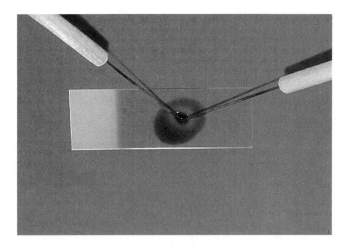

Figure 2–6. Teasing apart hyphae, tease mount.

TEASE MOUNT

Reagent Preparation
Lactophenol Cotton Blue—see LPCB wet mount

Procedure
1. Put one drop of LPCB stain on a glass slide.
2. With a flamed and cooled stiff wire inoculating needle, pick up a small portion of the fungal colony, cutting through the aerial and vegetative mycelium. Do not take the center or edge of the colony: the center is so old that hyphae may be sterile, while the edge is so young that reproductive structures may not yet have formed.
3. Place the fungal portion in the LPCB and, with a second needle, tease apart the hyphae so that they form a thin layer.
4. Put on a coverslip and press down hard to spread out the fungus. Examine under the microscope for reproductive structures.
5. For a permanent preparation, rim the edges of the coverslip with clear nail polish or Permount.

CELLOPHANE TAPE METHOD*

This works best with mature colonies growing on plates, rather than tubes, of media. Prepare a microscope slide with a drop of LPCB and set aside. Take a 2-inch piece of transparent cellophane tape, hold it between the fingers with the sticky side out, and touch the sticky side to the top of the fungal colony. Sporulation structures should stick to the tape. Now place the tape, sticky side down, on the microscope slide over the LPCB while stretching the tape and pressing both ends to attach it firmly to the slide. The tape acts as a coverglass. Examine under the microscope for fruiting structures. The advantage of this method is that it doesn't disturb the position of structures; however, it cannot be sealed for permanent storage.

An improved method (Rodriguez-Tudela and Aviles, 1991) uses a device which dispenses a thin layer of transparent adhesive to the surface of a cover glass (Pelikan Roll-Fix). Touch the sticky side of the cover glass to the top of the fungal colony, then place the cover glass (sticky side down) over a drop of LPCB on a microscope slide. This mount can be made permanent by sealing the edges with clear nail polish.

---

*If a dangerous, easily airborne organism such as *Coccidioides immitis* is suspected, do not use this technique.

SLIDE CULTURE METHOD   See box and Figures 2–7 through 2–14. The advantage of this method is that the fungal elements are grown and maintained in their original juxtaposition, thus making it easier to morphologically identify the organism. Also two mounts may be obtained from one culture. The disadvantages of this method are that it requires some technical expertise to set up the slide culture, and there is a waiting period for incubation of the slide culture in addition to incubation on the primary isolation medium before identifying the fungus. Also, cottony fungi, for example, the phylum Zygomycota, grow past the edges of the cover glass before forming reproductive structures.

SLIDE CULTURE METHOD

Procedure
1. Bring desired medium to room temperature. Bind together the ends of two applicator sticks with rubber bands. Break the sticks almost all the way through the middle so they form a V-shape. Alternatively, bend a glass rod or broken-off Pasteur pipette in a flame until it forms a V-shape, then cool. The sticks or glass rod serves as a platform on which to place the slide culture.
2. Place the sticks or rod in alcohol, dry, and put in the bottom of a sterile Petri dish.
3. Label a glass slide, dip in alcohol, flame dry, and set across the platform.
4. Place a 1-cm square block of potato dextrose agar (PDA) on the slide. This particular medium greatly enhances sporulation.
5. Using aseptic technique, inoculate a small piece of fungal colony from the primary isolation tube to one side of the agar block. When obtaining the inoculum, be sure to cut into the colony to get the vegetative as well as aerial growth. Do not take inoculum from the center or edge of the colony. Repeat this procedure for each side of the agar block.
6. Dip a glass coverslip (22 × 40 mm is recommended) in alcohol, flame, and place over the inoculated agar block. Press down lightly to ensure good contact between the agar and coverslip.
7. For moisture, pour about 5 mL of sterile distilled water into the bottom of the Petri dish. Cover the dish and set at room temperature to incubate. If all the water evaporates with time, add more.
8. The fungus will first grow on the sides of the agar, then out onto the slide and coverslip. Periodically examine the slide culture under a microscope. Look for fungal maturation, that is, characteristic reproductive structures.
9. When maturation is evident, remove the coverslip from the slide culture. Usually the agar block will come off with the coverslip; with a teasing needle, gently loosen the suction between agar and coverslip and decant the agar into disinfectant. Place the coverslip on a clean slide with one drop of LPCB.
10. If still remaining, remove the agar block from the bottom slide on the slide culture and drop into disinfectant. Put a drop of LPCB on this bottom slide and add a clean coverslip. Do not tamp down the coverslip, as this may jar conidia loose from the hyphae.
11. Gently heat the two LPCB preparations to release any trapped air bubbles and concentrate dye in the hyphae and reproductive structures. Observe the LPCB mounts under a microscope.
12. For permanent preparations, rim the coverslip edges with clear nail polish or Permount.

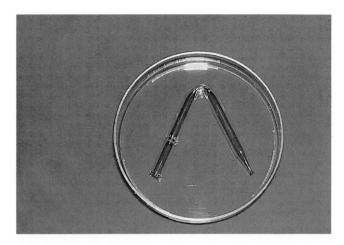

Figure 2–7. Glass rod in Petri dish, slide culture.

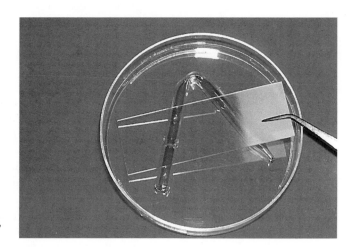

Figure 2–8. Glass slide over rod, slide culture.

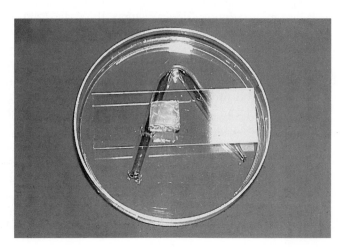

Figure 2–9. Agar block on slide, slide culture.

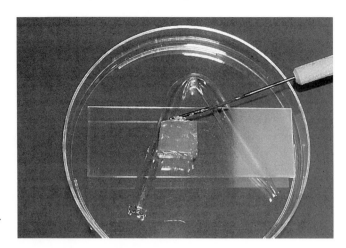

Figure 2–10. Inoculating agar block, slide culture.

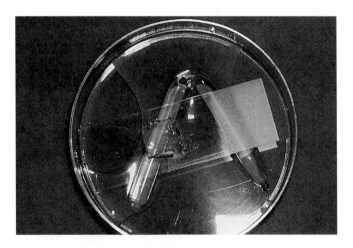

Figure 2–11. Flamed coverglass over agar and water in dish, slide culture.

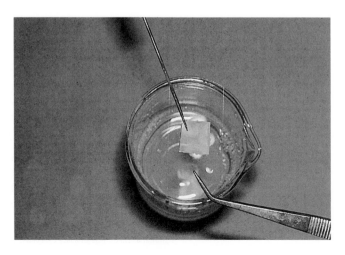

Figure 2–12. After incubation, agar block removed into disinfectant, slide culture.

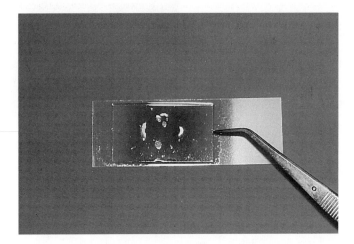

Figure 2–13. Coverslip put on slide with LPCB stain, slide culture.

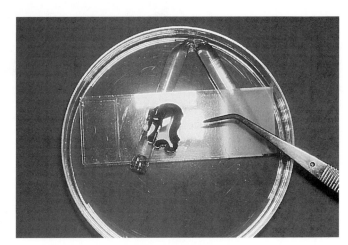

Figure 2–14. LPCB stain and coverslip put on slide from culture, slide culture.

MODIFIED SLIDE CULTURE METHOD This method uses water agar instead of distilled water for moisture. It also uses a cover glass on the bottom instead of a microscope slide (Harris 1986). (See box below.)

MODIFIED SLIDE CULTURE

Procedure:
1. Prepare water agar pour plates (20 g agar + 1 L distilled water) and store in refrigerator.
2. Flame and cool a cover glass; place the cover glass flat on top of water agar.
3. Put a cube of nutrient agar (potato dextrose agar) on the cover glass.
4. Using aseptic technique, inoculate each side of the agar block from the primary isolation colony.
5. Cover with another flamed and cooled cover glass.
6. Cover the dish and incubate.
7. When maturation is evident, remove the top cover glass and place on a microscope slide with a drop of LPCB.
8. Remove the agar block, discard, and mount the bottom cover glass on a microscope slide with a drop of LPCB.
9. For permanent preparations, seal edges of cover glass mounts with clear nail polish.

COVERSLIP SANDWICH TECHNIQUE See box and Figures 2–15 through 2–19. Several advantages of this technique are that more than two preparations may be made; each can be removed from the agar at different intervals; the set up is easier than for the slide culture; and the juxtaposition of reproductive structures to hyphae is almost as good as the slide culture method. The disadvantages are that the coverslip easily breaks while being inserted into the agar or when taken out, cottony fungi grow past the edges of the coverslip before forming reproductive structures, and there is a waiting period for incubation on the potato dextrose agar plate in addition to incubation on the primary isolation medium. Be cognizant that fungal elements formed on the coverslip beneath the agar are vegetative; only the aerial structures should be observed for mycologic identification.

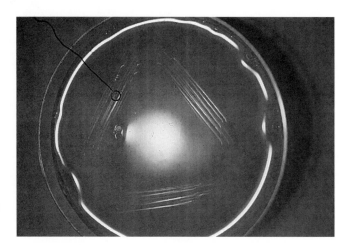

Figure 2–15. Streaks of fungus on potato dextrose agar (PDA), coverslip sandwich.

COVERSLIP SANDWICH TECHNIQUE

Medium Preparation
Potato dextrose agar (PDA)

Procedure
1. Bring PDA to room temperature. Streak small bits of fungal colony from the primary isolation medium onto the PDA surface. Be sure to take vegetative as well as aerial mycelium when obtaining the inoculum. Also, do not take fungus from the center or edge of the colony.
2. Dip a 22 × 22 mm glass coverslip in alcohol, flame-dry, and insert it into the agar at a 45-degree angle, over the fungal streaks. Repeat Step 2 with more glass coverslips.
3. Cover the plate and incubate at room temperature. At first the fungus will grow on the agar, then eventually up both sides of each coverslip.
4. When you think maturation is evident, gently remove one coverslip with forceps and place it on a slide containing a drop of LPCB. Add two to three drops more LPCB on top of the coverslip and put on a larger coverslip (24 × 40 mm works well). The 22 × 22 mm glass coverslip is now sandwiched between the larger one and the slide.
5. Observe under the microscope. Because there is fungal growth on both sides of the small coverslip, two different planes of focus are required to thoroughly examine the preparation.
6. If reproductive structures are present, remove the other glass coverslips from the PDA and mount them as in Step 4. If reproductive structures are not yet observed, reincubate the PDA plate and remove each glass coverslip when maturation occurs.
7. For permanent preparations, rim the large coverslips with clear nail polish or Permount.

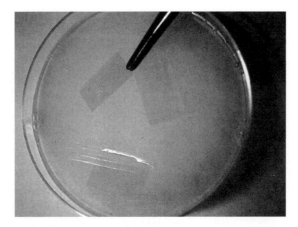

Figure 2–16. Coverslips inserted into streaks at 45-degree angle, coverslip sandwich.

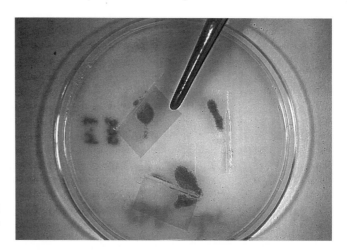

Figure 2–17. Coverslip removed when colony is mature, coverslip sandwich.

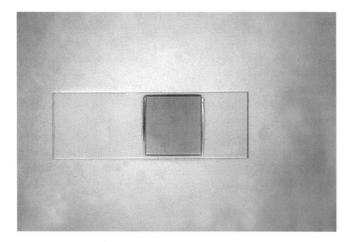

Figure 2–18. Coverslip on slide with LPCB stain, coverslip sandwich.

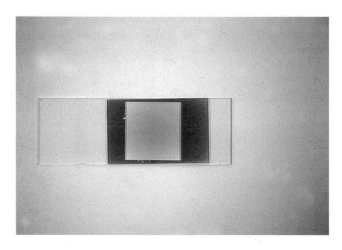

Figure 2–19. Second coverslip and LPCB stain over first coverslip, coverslip sandwich.

PROCEEDING TO SPECIFIC MODULES

Now that you know the specimen site, rate of growth, colonial morphology, and microscopic morphology, you may turn to specific modules for further differentiation of organisms.

GROWTH RATE	MICROSCOPIC	MODULE NUMBER AND TITLE
Rapid	Mold	3. Common Fungal Opportunists
Intermediate-slow	Mold	4. Superficial and Dermatophytic Fungi
Rapid	Yeast	5. Yeasts
Intermediate-slow	Mold, dimorphic fungus, funguslike bacterium	6. Organisms Causing Subcutaneous Mycoses
Intermediate-slow	Dimorphic fungus	7. Organisms Causing Systemic Mycoses

---

FINAL EXAM

1. Why should you not accept 24-hour collections on respiratory specimens?

2. Fill in the blanks: Two fungi that may be found in cerebrospinal fluid are _____ and _____.

3. Circle true or false:

   T   F   Fungal growth can be easily detected in blood culture bottles because the medium quickly becomes turbid.

4. Circle the correct answer: Lactophenol cotton blue stains the chitin/keratin in fungal cell walls.

5. One role of the mycology laboratory is to isolate fungi as quickly as possible, while keeping down costs. In your opinion, what is the best general incubation temperature for primary fungal cultures? Justify your answer.

6. List the advantages and disadvantages of the following:
   A. Tease Mount

   B. Slide Culture/Modified Slide Culture

C. Coverslip Sandwich

7. How do specimen site, colonial morphology, and general microscopic morphology (i.e., mold, yeast, dimorphic fungus, or funguslike bacteria) aid in identification?

STOP HERE UNTIL YOU HAVE COMPLETED THE ANSWERS.
Look up the answers in the back of the book. If you missed more than one of them, go back and repeat this module. Correctly complete any missed questions before proceeding.

SUPPLEMENTAL RATIONALE

SKIN TESTS

An extract of the antigen (known fungus) is injected into the patient's skin. After 24 to 48 hours, the site is observed for **erythema** (redness) and swelling, and measured for **induration** (hardness). This reaction is caused by a delayed hypersensitivity in patients who have been previously exposed to the antigen. Skin tests are usually performed in patients suspected of having histoplasmosis, blastomycosis, or coccidioidomycosis. Since there is cross reactivity between these three antigens, all three are injected at the same time but at different sites. More than one site may give hardness and redness; however, the one with induration of 5 mm or more in diameter is the organism the patient was previously exposed to.

Since the skin will test positive years after the patient came in contact with the antigen, the skin test is of limited use in diagnosis of present active infection. Also the skin test may be negative in the acute stage of infection (no immunologic response synthesized yet), in patients who are immunosuppressed, or in patients who have overwhelming fungal infection. Do not administer a skin test before taking blood for other serologic studies. Injected skin test antigen will stimulate antibody production, which may give a false-positive reaction in serologic procedures.

SEROMYCOLOGY

Tests to detect fungal antibody from serum include immunodiffusion, indirect latex agglutination, complement fixation, indirect immunofluorescence, counterimmunoelectrophoresis, and enzyme-linked immunosorbent assay (ELISA). A fourfold rise in titer of paired sera drawn 2 to 3 weeks apart increases sensitivity; however, the delay in diagnosis diminishes the usefulness of the procedure. Some of the newer methods include immunodiffusion for subcutaneous zygomycosis (Kaufman et al. 1990), ELISA for *H. capsulatum* (Zimmerman et al. 1990), enzyme immunoassay for *P. brasiliensis* IgM and IgG (Camargo et al. 1994), and Premier enzyme immunoassay (Meridian Diagnostics) for *C. immitis* IgM and IgG (Kaufman et al. 1995; Martins et al. 1995). The bioMerieux test for IgM and IgG antibody in disseminated candidiasis is 100% sensitive and 100% specific (Gutierrez et al. 1993).

Tests to detect fungal antigen may use specimen directly (e.g., cryptococcal antigen from serum or CSF), or bits of fungal colony once isolated (e.g., exoantigen testing of systemic pathogens by immunodiffusion). Techniques include immunodiffusion/exoantigen, indirect reverse latex agglutination, direct fluorescent antibody, enzyme immunoassay, and avidin-biotin ELISA. Exoantigen tests are 100% specific for *B. dermatitidis*, *C. immitis*, and *P. brasiliensis* within 48 to 72 hours (Padhye et al. 1994).

Kits to detect *Candida* mannan polysaccharide antigen in specimens are Cand-Tec latex agglutination (Ramco Labs), Directogen (Becton Dickinson), and Pastorex (Sanofi Diagnostics Pasteur). Under optimal conditions (serum drawn within 24 hours of diagnosis of invasive candidiasis), Cand-Tec is 57% sensitive (Lemieux et al. 1990). Directogen is (+) in 80% of true positive specimens, but also falsely (+) in 10% (Gutierrez et al. 1993). Pastorex was (−) in all true positive specimens in one study (Gutierrez et al. 1993). Other noncommercial methods for detecting *Candida* antigen in patient specimens are dot immunobinding (Riboli 1993), ELISA (Lemieux et al. 1990), and avidin-biotin enzyme immunoassay (Nakamura et al. 1991). Additionally, there are nonimmunologic methods for determining *C. albicans* metabolite (arabinitol) from specimens.

Cryptococcal antigen kits detect fungal antigen in clinical specimens: Calas-LA latex agglutination (Meridian Diagnostics), Crypto-LA latex agglutination (International Biological Labs), Myco-Immune latex agglutination (American Micro-Scan), Immy Latex-Crypto Antigen (Immuno-Mycologics), monoclonal antibody based Crypto-Lex latex agglutination (Trinity Labs), and Premier cryptococcal antigen enzyme immunoassay (Meridian Diagnostics). These kits are capable of detecting as little as 20 to 30 nanograms of antigen per milliliter of serum or cerebrospinal fluid. All latex kits require heat inactivation to reduce nonspecific interference and inactivate complement. Also pretreat serum and CSF (Crypto-LA) or just serum (Calas-LA) with pronase to increase antigen titer and convert some (−) specimens to true (+) (Hamilton et al. 1991). All the kits give comparable CSF sensitivities (93 to 100%) and specificities (93 to 98%). However the pronase-pretreated serum latex methods and the enzyme immunoassay method give greater sensitivities (97%) than the non-pronase methods (83%). Specificity for serum was approximately the same with all kits (93 to 100%) (Tanner et al. 1994; Kiska et al. 1994). False positives on cryptococcal antigen testing include: *Trichosporon* infection (Melcher et al. 1991), collagen vascular disease, malignancy, rheumatoid arthritis, and syneresis fluid (surface condensation from agar plates) (Heelan et al. 1991). Crypto-LA did give a false (+) with syneresis fluid, but not with the other factors; whereas Premier EIA gave no false (+) results with any of the factors (Engler and Shea 1994). Some false positives can be eliminated by pretreatment with 2-B-mercaptoethanol (Whittier et al. 1994).

Newer developments in fungal antigen testing are an exoantigen immunodiffusion test for identifying *Exophiala* (Standard et al. 1991), the Pastorex *Aspergillus* kit which uses monoclonal antibody to detect *Aspergillus* antigen in patient serum (Kappe and Schulze-Berge 1993), and an immunoradiometric assay for *P. brasiliensis* antigens in serum (deFatima Ferreira-da-Cruz et al. 1991).

DNA TESTING DNA probes are extremely useful for quickly identifying clinical isolates of slower growing fungi. A commercially available system (AccuProbe, made by GenProbe) exists for *H. capsulatum*, *B. dermatitidis*, *C. immitis*, and *C. neoformans*.

A known luminescent-labelled, single-stranded DNA probe to the organism in question is allowed to hybridize with unknown ribosomal RNA from a sonicated culture. If the fungus in question is present, the fungal rRNA will combine with probe DNA and luminesce when placed in a luminometer.

This method is the most sensitive and specific of any on the market (Huffnagle and Gander 1993; Stockman et al. 1993; Padhye et al. 1994). The probes to *H. capsulatum*, *C. neoformans*, and *C. immitis* are 100% sensitive and 100% specific. The *B. dermatitidis* AccuProbe is 97.3% sensitive, but 10 of 17 *P. brasiliensis* isolates were identified as *B. dermatitidis*.

Another technique which shows great promise is the polymerase chain reaction (PCR); however, no commercial kits are yet available. This can be performed on clinical specimens with suspected fungi, or on fungal isolates. PCR can detect as little as one strand of fungal DNA in a specimen, as the technique amplifies DNA a millionfold. Another method such as restriction enzyme analysis then identifies the fungus. The problem is that these techniques may be actually too sensitive. They have been used to detect

Aspergillus in respiratory specimens, but about 25% of negative controls give positive results, probably from *Aspergillus* colonization (Spreadbury et al. 1993; Melchers et al. 1994; Bretagne et al. 1995). *Candida* has been isolated from blood specimens in a similar manner, but again there was the problem of contamination with *Candida* skin flora from when the blood was drawn (Miyakawa et al. 1993; Holmes et al. 1994; Fujita et al. 1995). Another study (Hopfer et al. 1993) was able to break down unknown fungi into five groups (*Candida, Cryptococcus* and *Trichosporon, Aspergillus,* zygomycetes, and dimorphs) with more research needed to specifically identify the organisms.

CULTURE PRESERVATION

The easiest way to maintain stock fungal cultures is the distilled water method of Castellani (Castellani 1939; Castellani 1963). After growth and sporulation of the fungus on solid medium (Sabouraud's or potato dextrose agar), place 2 to 3 mL of sterile distilled water over the culture. Scrape the sporulating structures into the water with a sterile wire loop or pipette tip. Aspirate the water with a sterile pipette and transfer to a sterile screw-capped tube. Tighten the cap and store at room temperature or in the refrigerator. Overall survival is 97% for the first 5 years; however, *Candida krusei* and *Saccharomyces cerevisiae* may not survive (Odds 1991).

Other techniques include freezing, lyophilization, and oil overlay. See Kwon-Chung and Bennett (Kwon-Chung and Bennett 1992) for further details.

THERAPY FOR MYCOSES

In the past, treatment of systemic fungal infections required amphotericin B (Amp B), with its set of toxic renal effects. Now newer fungicidal agents are being evaluated in Europe, and many systemic fungistatic agents (fluorocytosine, azoles) are available in the United States (Richardson and Warnock 1993; Kwon-Chung and Bennett 1992). (see Chart 2–5.)

Agents

Polyene Macrolides. These agents (Amp B, Nystatin) are inserted into the fungal membrane phospholipid, creating pores that increase membrane permeability, allowing small molecules to leak out.

Intravenous Amp B remains the empiric therapy for suspected systemic fungemia in neutropenic patients. Its spectrum of activity includes candidiasis, cryptococcosis, histoplasmosis, blastomycosis, paracoccidioidomycosis, coccidioidomycosis, aspergillosis, extracutaneous sporotrichosis, and zygomycosis. The most common side effects are renal failure, hypokalemia, hypomagnesemia, and anemia. These are ameliorated by heavy hydration with normal saline before and after the antibiotic, and potassium/magnesium supplements. Organisms now becoming resistant to Amp B are *T. beigelii, C. tropicalis, C. lusitaniae, C. guillermondii,* and *C. parapsilosis* (Walsh et al. 1990)

Nystatin (Mycostatin, Nilstat) is used orally, vaginally, or topically for *Candida.* Because it is not given intravenously, there are virtually no side effects. Unfortunately it is not very potent; thus it must be given for a prolonged period of time to show efficacy.

Pyrimidine Analogues. 5-Fluorocytosine (5-FC) is a pyrimidine analogue, which incorporates into RNA to cause production of a nonsense protein. Otherwise, it can convert into a potent thymidylate synthetase inhibitor, which stops DNA production. It has been used for candidiasis, cryptococcosis, and chromoblastomycosis. Unfortunately, organisms quickly develop resistance.

5-FC is synergistic with Amp B against most systemic *Candida* and *C. neoformans,* allowing a lesser dose of Amp B, and lessening development of resistance.

5-FC is also synergistic with fluconazole on *C. albicans,* giving an effect lasting 2.5 hours longer per dose than either agent alone (Mikami et al. 1992).

Azole Antifungals. These include clotrimazole (Lotrimin), miconazole (Micatin, Monistat), ketoconazole (Nizoral), itraconazole (Sporanox), and fluconazole (Diflucan). These can be given topically, orally, or intravenously, depending on the azole derivative. Azoles bind to the heme portion of cytochrome P450 to interfere with mixed oxidase functions. They also block formation of ergosterol in the fungal cell membrane, inhibit-

CHART 2–5. ANTIFUNGAL DRUGS AND THE DISEASES THEY TREAT

	Polyene; Macrolides		Pyrimidine analogue	Azoles					Griseofulvin	Allylamine
	Amphotericin B	Nystatin	5-Fluorocytosine	Clotrimazole	Miconazole	Ketoconazole	Itraconazole	Fluconazole	Griseofulvin	Terbinafine
Mode of administration:	T/PO/IV*	T/PO	PO	T/PO	T/PO/IV	T/PO	PO	PO/IV	PO	T/PO
Disease:										
Aspergillosis	+				+	–	+	–		
Blastomycosis	+				+	+	+	+	–	
Candidiasis	+	+	+ many resis.	+	+	+	+	mod		fungistatic
Chromoblastomycosis (*C. carrionii, Fonsecaea, P. verrucosa*)	some		+							
Coccidioidomycosis	+				+	+	+	+		
Cryptococcosis	+		+ many resis.		+		+	+		
Dermatophytosis (*Trichophyton, Microsporum, Epidermophyton*)				+	+	+	+	+	+	+
Histoplasmosis	+				+	+	+	+		
Paracoccidioidomycosis	+				+	+	+	+		
Pityriasis	some		–	+	+		+			
Infection due to *Scedosporium apiospermium*	–				+	–		–	–	–
Zygomycosis	some									

*T = topical, PO = oral, IV= intravenous.

ing growth. While usually fungistatic, some topical preparations can be fungicidal. Azoles are useful for candidiasis, cryptococcosis, coccidioidomycosis, blastomycosis, histoplasmosis, scedosporiosis, pityriasis versicolor, dermatophytosis (ringworm), aspergillosis, and sporotrichosis.

Prophylaxis for candidiasis in immunosuppressed transplant patients is oral ketoconazole (or itraconazole, because of its less toxic side effects). Both agents cause increased cyclosporin levels (cyclosporin is used as an immunosuppressive to prevent graft rejection); thus a lesser dose of cyclosporin may successfully be used along with the azole to prevent both graft rejection and mycotic infection.

Fluconazole does not raise cyclosporin levels. It is the agent of choice for oral or esophageal candidiasis in AIDS patients because it's more reliably absorbed despite AIDS gastropathy. Unfortunately, though, resistant strains are surfacing (Pfaller et al. 1994; Millon et al. 1994). With fluconazole-resistant thrush in AIDS patients, use oral Amp B or itraconazole (Dewsnup and Stevens 1994; Ruhnke et al. 1994). Fluconazole has been used successfully to treat cryptococcal meningitis in African AIDS patients, with a clinical cure of 63% and negative culture after 60 to 90 days of therapy in 76% of patients (Laroche et al. 1992). Unfortunately, in immunocompromised or granulocytopenic patients, fluconazole has been shown to obscure the onset of aspergillosis (Kappe et al. 1993).

Patients with chronic mucocutaneous candidiasis have hyperkeratotic lesions that do not respond to topical therapy; thus oral ketoconazole or itraconazole are the agents of choice.

Griseofulvin. This drug works by interaction with polymerized microtubules and disruption of the mitotic spindle. It is fungicidal. Griseofulvin is taken orally for treatment of dermatophytosis (*Trichophyton, Microsporum,* and *Epidermophyton*), and must be continued until the infected hair, nail, or skin has completely grown out and been replaced.

Allylamines. Topical naftifine (Naftin) and oral/topical terbinafine (Lamisil) act by inhibiting squalene epoxidase, an essential step in ergosterol synthesis. Both are used for dermatophytosis.

STUDY QUESTIONS

1. All of the following are true concerning skin tests for blastomycosis, histoplasmosis, and coccidioidomycosis *except:*

    A. Since all three antigens cross-react, the one that produces 5 mm or more of hardness is the positive test.

    B. Perform the skin tests before taking blood for serology.

    C. Overwhelming fungal infection may produce a negative skin test to the corresponding antigen.

    D. Skin tests remain positive years after active infection.

    E. Immunologically suppressed patients may not give a positive test, even in active infection.

2. State if the following serologic methods detect fungal antigen, fungal antibody, or both.

    A. Immunodiffusion _____

    B. Latex agglutination _____

    C. Direct fluorescent antibody _____

    D. ELISA _____

3. On cryptococcal antigen testing, list three causes of false-positive results, and one way to decrease them.

4. What is the principle behind the DNA probe procedure?

5. Give four methods for fungal stock culture preservation.

   1. _____

   2. _____

   3. _____

   4. _____

6. List the five basic classes of antifungal agents and give one example of each. Discuss which mycoses (systemic, dermatophytic, yeast, subcutaneous) each class usually treats.

7. Discuss problems with successful antifungal treatment of immunocompromised patients.

STOP HERE UNTIL YOU HAVE COMPLETED THE QUESTIONS.

Look up the answers in the back of the book. If you missed more than two, go back and repeat the supplemental rationale portion of this module. Correctly complete any missed questions.

Common Fungal Opportunists

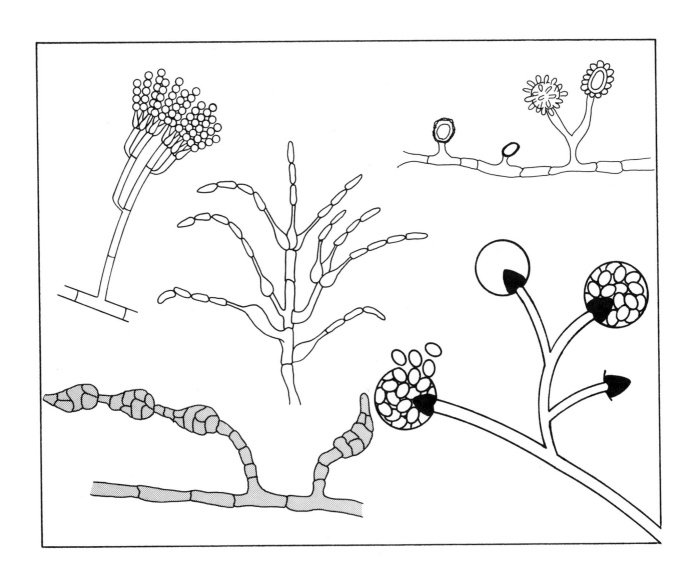

MODULE

3

Common Fungal Opportunists

PREREQUISITES

The learner must possess a good background knowledge in clinical microbiology and must have finished Module 1, Basics of Mycology, and Module 2, Laboratory Procedures for Fungal Culture and Isolation.

BEHAVIORAL OBJECTIVES

Upon completion of this module, the learner should be able to:

1   Define:
Saprobe
Opportunistic pathogen   Dematiaceous
Hyaline   Penicillus

2   Discuss at least five common properties of fungal opportunists.

3   From fungal colonies and microscopic preparations, recognize the following:
Aseptate Opportunists   *Epicoccum* sp.
Absidia sp.   *Nigrospora* sp.
Apophysomyces sp.   *Acremonium* sp.
Cunninghamella sp.   *Aspergillus* sp., especially *A. fumigatus*
Mucor sp.   *Chrysosporium* sp.
Rhizopus sp.   *Fusarium* sp.
Saksenaea sp.   *Gliocladium* sp.
Syncephalastrum sp.   *Penicillium* sp.
Septate Opportunists   *Paecilomyces* sp.
Alternaria sp.   *Scopulariopsis* sp.
Cladosporium sp.   *Sepedonium* sp.
Aureobasidium sp.   *Ulocladium* sp.
Bipolaris sp.   *Stemphylium* sp.
Curvularia sp.   Shield cells
Exserohilum sp.   Foot cells of *Aspergillus* and *Fusarium*

4   Given a fungal microscopic preparation, classify the organism as aseptate or septate, and if septate, categorize as hyaline or dematiaceous.

5   Compare and contrast the microscopic features of *Absidia* sp., *Mucor* sp., *Rhizopus* sp., *Apophysomyces* sp., *Cunninghamella* sp., and *Saksenaea* sp.

6   Describe at least two ways to differentiate the similar-appearing dark molds *Epicoccum*, *Ulocladium*, and *Stemphylium*.

7   Contrast the poroconidial arrangement of *Curvularia*, *Bipolaris*, *Helminthosporium*, and *Exserohilum* sp.

75

8 Discuss ways to distinguish *Acremonium* from the subcutaneous pathogen *Sporothrix schenckii.*

9 Compare and contrast the opportunists *Chrysosporium* and *Sepedonium* with the subcutaneous disease producer *Scedosporium apiospermum* and the systemic pathogens *Histoplasma capsulatum* and *Blastomyces dermatitidis.*

10 List three microscopic differences between *Aspergillus* sp. and the similar-appearing organism, *Syncephalastrum* sp.

11 From microscopic mounts and cultural characteristics, differentiate *Aspergillus fumigatus* from other *Aspergillus* species.

12 Compare and contrast colonial and microscopic morphology of *Penicillium* sp., *Paecilomyces* sp., *Gliocladium* sp., and *Scopulariopsis* sp.

13 List two differences between *Fusarium* sp. and *Cylindrocarpon* sp.

14 Briefly elaborate on the symptoms for these opportunistic mycoses:

Aspergillosis	Penicilliosis
Keratomycosis	Sinusitis
Otomycosis	Zygomycosis

Include predisposing factors, basis for etiologic significance, and three causative agents for each.

CONTENT OUTLINE

I. Introduction
II. Common properties of fungal opportunists
  A. Rapid-growing
  B. Saprobic and airborne
  C. Normally inhaled
  D. Opportunistic pathogens
  E. Laboratory diagnosis
III. Aseptate opportunists
  A. Terminal vesicle absent
    1. *Absidia* species
    2. *Apophysomyces* species
    3. *Mucor* species
    4. *Rhizopus* species
    5. *Saksenaea* species
  B. Terminal vesicle present
    1. *Cunninghamella* species
    2. *Syncephalastrum* species
  C. Zygomycosis
  D. Study questions
IV. Septate opportunists
  A. Dematiaceous opportunists
    1. *Alternaria* species
    2. *Aureobasidium* species
    3. *Bipolaris* species
    4. *Cladosporium (Hormodendrum)* species

    5. *Curvularia* species
    6. *Exserohilum* species
    7. *Epicoccum* species
    8. *Nigrospora* species
    9. Study questions
  B. Hyaline opportunists
    1. *Acremonium (Cephalosporium)* species
    2. *Aspergillus* species
    3. *Chrysosporium* species
    4. *Fusarium* species
    5. *Gliocladium* species
    6. *Paecilomyces* species
    7. *Penicillium* species
    8. *Scopulariopsis* species
    9. *Sepedonium* species
    10. Study questions
  C. Opportunistic mycoses
    1. Aspergillosis
    2. Penicilliosis
    3. Keratomycosis
    4. Otomycosis
    5. Sinusitis
V. Final Exam

FOLLOW-UP ACTIVITIES

1 Students may identify unknown organisms by colonial and microscopic appearance.
2 Students may open up a sterile Sabouraud dextrose agar plate in a location of their choice (subway station, shower stall, or so forth) and expose the plate for 5 minutes. Incubate the plate at room temperature and observe which opportunists grow.

REFERENCES

Bearer, EA, et al: Cutaneous zygomycosis caused by *Saksenaea vasiformis* in a diabetic patient. J Clin Microbiol 32:1823, 1994.

Castro, LGM, et al: Hyalohyphomycosis by *Paecilomyces lilacinus* in a renal transplant patient and a review of human *Paecilomyces* species infection. J Med Vet Mycol 28:15, 1990.

Cody, DT, et al: Allergic fungal sinusitis: the Mayo Clinic experience. Laryngoscope 104:1074, 1994.

Deng, Z and Connor, DH: Progressive disseminated penicilliosis caused by *Penicillium marneffei*. Am J Clin Pathol 84:323, 1985.

Eaton, ME, et al: Osteomyelitis of the sternum caused by *Apophysomyces elegans*. J Clin Microbiol 32:2827, 1994.

Friedman, GC, et al: Allergic fungal sinusitis, report of three cases associated with dematiaceous fungi. Am J Clin Pathol 96:368, 1991.

Gene, J, et al: Cutaneous phaeohyphomycosis caused by *Alternaria longipes* in an immunosuppressed patient. J Clin Microbiol 33:2774, 1995.

Hopwood, V, et al: Primary cutaneous zygomycosis due to *Absidia corymbifera* in a patient with AIDS. J Med Vet Mycol 30:399, 1992.

Koneman, EW, et al: Practical Laboratory Mycology, ed 3. Williams & Wilkins, Baltimore, 1985.

Kwon-Chung, KJ and Bennett, JE: Medical Mycology. Lea & Febiger, Philadelphia, 1992.

Lakshmi, V, et al: Zygomycotic necrotizing fasciitis caused by *Apophysomyces elegans*. J Clin Microbiol 31:1368, 1993.

Larone, DH: Medically Important Fungi, ed 3. ASM Press, Washington, DC, 1995.

Leenders, A, et al: Molecular epidemiology of apparent outbreak of invasive aspergillosis in a hematology ward. J Clin Microbiol 34:345, 1996.

Loveless, MD, et al: Mixed invasive infection with *Alternaria* species and *Curvularia* species. Am J Clin Pathol 76:491, 1981.

McGinnis, MR: Laboratory Handbook of Medical Mycology. Academic Press, New York, 1980.

McGinnis, MR, et al: Emerging agents of phaeohyphomycosis: pathogenic species of *Bipolaris* and *Exserohilum*. J Clin Microbiol 24:250, 1986.

Meis, JFGM, et al: Severe osteomyelitis due to the zygomycete *Apophysomyces elegans*. J Clin Microbiol 32:3078, 1994.

Melcher, GP, et al: Disseminated hyalohyphomycosis caused by a novel human pathogen, *Fusarium napiforme*. J Clin Microbiol 31:1461, 1993.

Mowbray, DN, et al: Disseminated *Fusarium solani* infection with cutaneous nodules in a bone marrow transplant patient. Int J Dermatol 27:698, 1988.

Nalesnik, MA, et al: Significance of *Aspergillus* species isolated from respiratory secretions in the diagnosis of invasive pulmonary aspergillosis. J Clin Microbiol 11:370, 1980.

Padhye, AA and Ajello, L: Simple method of inducing sporulation by *Apophysomyces elegans* and *Saksenaea vasiformis*. J Clin Microbiol 26:1861, 1988.

Padhye, AA, et al: Phaeohyphomycosis of the nasal sinuses caused by a new species of *Exserohilum*. J Clin Microbiol 24:245, 1986.

Panke, TW, et al: Infection of a burn wound by *Aspergillus niger*. Am J Clin Pathol 73:230, 1979.

Perfect, JR, et al: Uncommon invasive fungal pathogens in the acquired immunodeficiency syndrome. J Med Vet Mycol 31:175, 1993.

Peto, TEA, et al: Systemic mycosis due to *Penicillium marneffei* in a patient with antibody to human immunodeficiency virus. J Infect 16:285, 1988.

Pierce, PF, et al: *Saksenaea vasiformis* osteomyelitis. J Clin Microbiol 25:933, 1987.

Schell, WA: Oculomycosis caused by dematiaceous fungi. Proceedings of the VI International Conference on the Mycoses, Pan American Health Organization, Washington, DC, 1986.

Singh, SM, et al: Ungual and cutaneous phaeohyphomycosis caused by *Alternaria alternata* and *Alternaria chlamydospora*. J Med Vet Mycol 28:275, 1990.

Summerbell, RC, et al: *Fusarium proliferatum* as an agent of disseminated infection in an immunosuppressed patient. J Clin Microbiol 26:82, 1988.

Thomas, PA: Mycotic keratitis—an underestimated mycosis. J Med Vet Mycol 32:235, 1994.

Weitzman, I, et al: *Mucor ramosissimus* Samutsevitsch isolated from a thigh lesion. J Clin Microbiol 31:2523, 1993.

West, BC, et al: Mucormycosis caused by *Rhizopus microsporus* var. *microsporus*: cellulitis in the leg of a diabetic patient cured by amputation. J Clin Microbiol 33:3341, 1995.

INTRODUCTION This module discusses some of the more common genera of fungal opportunists that the practicing medical mycologist may encounter. There are many more known opportunists, but it is beyond the scope of this module to present them all.

Opportunists will be seen very often in routine fungal cultures, and it is therefore important to be able to identify and differentiate them from the regularly **pathogenic** (disease producing) fungi, which are presented in Modules 4 through 7.

COMMON PROPERTIES OF FUNGAL OPPORTUNISTS

There are a number of generalizations that can be made regarding fungal opportunists.

RAPID-GROWING

Most are rapid growers, forming mature colonies in 4 or 5 days.

SAPROBIC AND AIRBORNE

They are **saprobic,** living on decaying organic matter in the soil, and sometimes become airborne.

NORMALLY INHALED

Since we constantly inhale the conidia of fungal opportunists, routine cultures of sputum and other respiratory secretions may normally yield a few colonies of these organisms. Also, since the conidia are in the air, they may contaminate the skin as well as laboratory cultures.

OPPORTUNISTIC PATHOGENS

Usually these organisms are nonpathogenic. However, they act as **opportunistic pathogens.** When the patient is debilitated in some way, as from illness or especially from immunosuppressive drugs, these common organisms may multiply and cause disease, often with fatal consequences.

LABORATORY DIAGNOSIS

In order to isolate an opportunist, be sure to inoculate media free of antibiotics, since the drugs inhibit these fungi. Because they are so common in the environment, opportunistic pathogens must be repeatedly isolated in large numbers from cultured specimens of the patient, or from normally sterile sites, to be considered the causative agent of the disease. Since fungal opportunists are differentiated on the basis of their microscopic morphology, isolates should be transferred to media such as potato dextrose or corn meal agar to enhance formation of characteristic conidia.

ASEPTATE OPPORTUNISTS

All aseptate fungi, those with hyphae that usually do not contain cross-walls, fall into the taxonomic phylum Zygomycota. A few of the more important Zygomycetes that act as opportunistic pathogens follow. Key identifying features are capitalized. Also, Chart 3-1 on pages 80 and 81 may be helpful.

TERMINAL VESICLE ABSENT

The sporangiophores of these organisms end in columellae around which sporangia form.

Absidia Species (Figs. 3–1 and 3–2)

Culture: On SABHI agar at room temperature, a woolly gray colony rapidly matures (see Color Plate 14). The reverse side of the colony is colorless.

Microscopic: The mycelium is usually ASEPTATE, with BRANCHING SPORANGIO-PHORES BETWEEN the **RHIZOIDS** (rootlike hyphae) on the **STOLONS** (interconnecting runners). There is a slight swelling below the columella, and sporangia are PEAR-SHAPED. When the sporangial wall dissolves, a collarette remains at the base of the columella.

Pathogenicity: Absidia may cause zygomycosis and keratomycosis. See later sections of this module for descriptions of these diseases.

Apophysomyces Species (Figs. 3–3 and 3–4)

Culture: On SABHI agar at room temperature, cottony white colonies may mature rapidly, becoming off-white to yellow with age. *Apophysomyces* sp. is thermo-tolerant, growing at temperatures up to 42 °C.

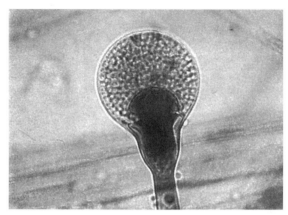

Figure 3–1. *Absidia* sp., lactophenol cotton blue (LPCB) stain (magnification ×450).

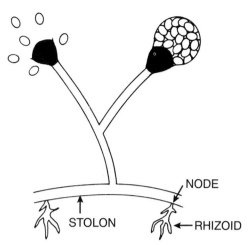

Figure 3–2. *Absidia* sp.

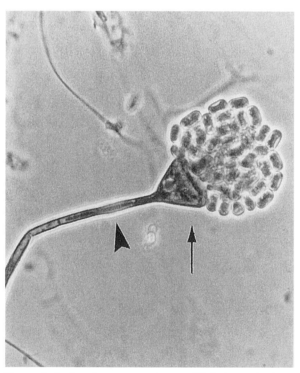

Figure 3–3. *Apophysomyces elegans* (CDC B-5049) after 7 days' incubation in distilled water–yeast extract medium at 37°C (magnification ×560). (From Eaton, et al: J Clin Microbiol 1994, with permission.)

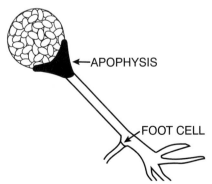

Figure 3–4. *Apophysomyces* sp.

CHART 3–1. KEY TO IDENTIFICATION OF CLINICALLY IMPORTANT ZYGOMYCOTA*

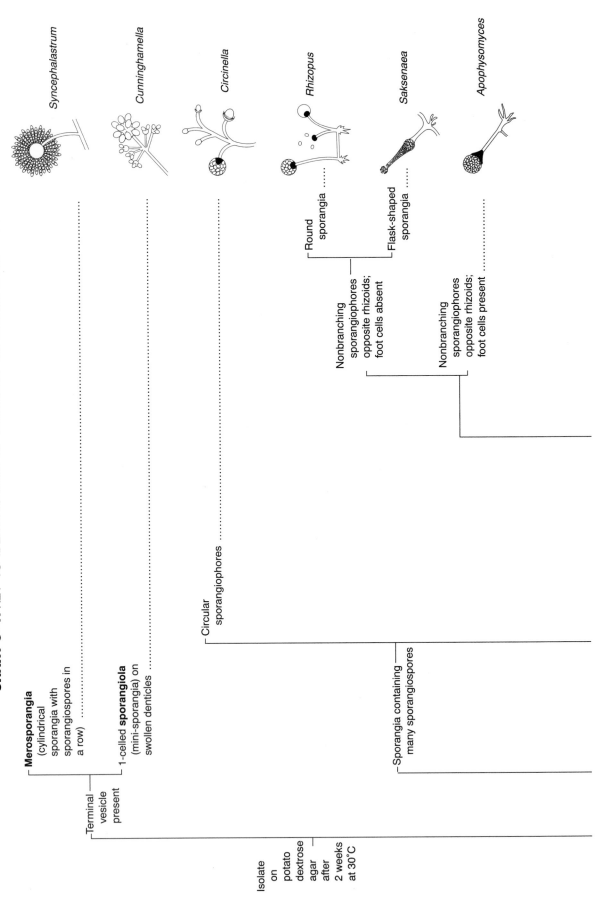

Isolate on potato dextrose agar after 2 weeks at 30°C

Terminal vesicle present

Merosporangia (cylindrical sporangia with sporangiospores in a row) .... *Syncephalastrum*

1-celled **sporangiola** (mini-sporangia) on swollen denticles .... *Cunninghamella*

Circular sporangiophores .... *Circinella*

Sporangia containing many sporangiospores

Nonbranching sporangiophores opposite rhizoids; foot cells absent

Round sporangia .... *Rhizopus*

Flask-shaped sporangia .... *Saksenaea*

Nonbranching sporangiophores opposite rhizoids; foot cells present .... *Apophysomyces*

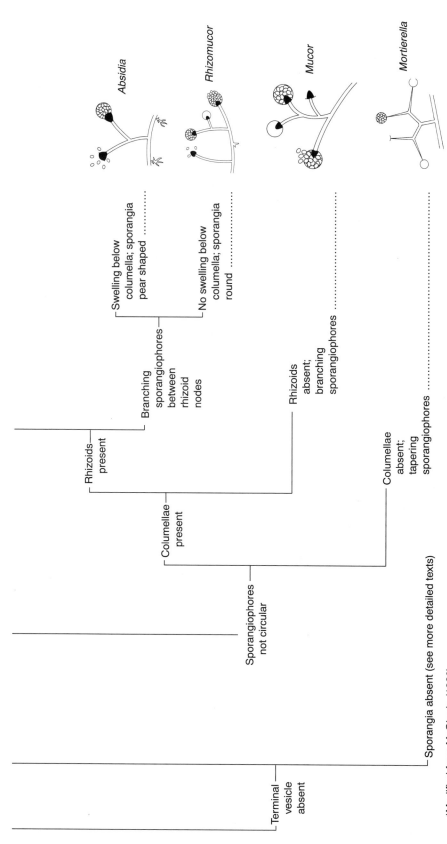

Modified from McGinnis (1980).

Microscopic: On SABHI agar, or even on nutritionally deficient media such as corn meal or potato dextrose agar, at room temperature, the hyphae usually fail to sporulate. To induce sporulation, Padhye and Ajello (1988) suggest aseptically transferring blocks of SABHI agar inoculated with fungus to tubes of sterile distilled water—10% yeast extract medium (without hair) used for the in vitro hair perforation test (see page 134), and incubating at 37°C for 10 to 14 days. Under these conditions, unbranched SPORAN-GIOPHORES with **FOOT CELLS** (bases) and funnel-shaped **APOPHYSES** (swollen columellae) may be seen. Thin-walled RHIZOIDS may form opposite the sporangiophores. SPORANGIA are pyriform and contain oblong SPORANGIOSPORES.

Pathogenicity: Apophysomyces is a cause of zygomycosis.

Mucor Species
(Figs. 3–5 and 3–6)

Culture: On SABHI agar at room temperature, a white, fluffy mycelium quickly forms (see Color Plate 15). It becomes gray to brown with age.

Microscopic: The mycelium is usually ASEPTATE. Single or BRANCHING SPORANGIO-PHORES support round, spore-filled sporangia. Sometimes empty sporangial sacs or bare columellae with collarettes may be seen. The columella is variable in shape and light to pigmented in color. NO RHIZOIDS OR STOLONS are present.

Pathogenicity: Mucor may cause zygomycosis, **otomycosis** (ear infection), and allergies.

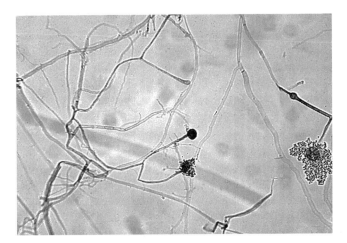

Figure 3–5. *Mucor* sp., LPCB stain (magnification ×100).

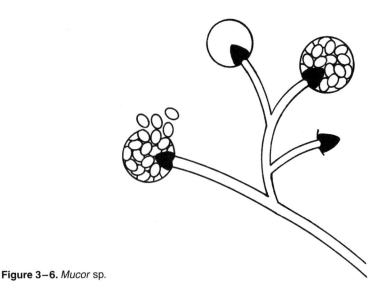

Figure 3–6. *Mucor* sp.

Rhizopus Species
(Figs. 3–7 and 3–8)

Culture: On SABHI agar at room temperature, white, dense, cottony aerial hyphae rapidly form, which later become dotted with brown or black sporangia (see Color Plate 3).

Microscopic: The hyphae are usually ASEPTATE. UNBRANCHED SPORANGIOPHORES arise OPPOSITE RHIZOIDS at the nodes, and each sporangiophore supports a round spore-filled sporangium with a flattened base. Sometimes the sporangia are completely black, or they may be empty. When the sporangial wall dissolves, a bare hemispherical columella without a collarette is observed. STOLONS connect the groups of rhizoids with each other.

Pathogenicity: Rhizopus causes zygomycosis and otomycosis.

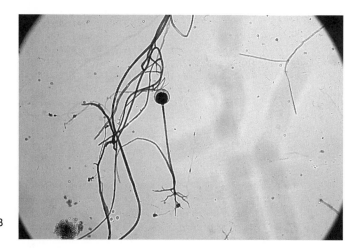

Figure 3–7. *Rhizopus* sp., LPCB stain (magnification ×100).

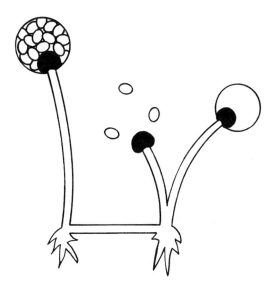

Figure 3–8. *Rhizopus* sp.

Saksenaea Species
(Figs. 3−9 and 3−10)

Culture: On SABHI agar at room temperature, rapidly growing woolly white colonies are seen.

Microscopic: The broad hyphae are usually ASEPTATE to sparsely septate and branched. On blocks of SABHI agar growing in distilled water-yeast extract medium at 37°C, typical FLASK-SHAPED SPORANGIA are observed that produce smooth, elongated sporangiospores. RHIZOIDS are produced opposite the sporangiophores.

Pathogenicity: Saksenaea may cause zygomycosis and osteomyelitis.

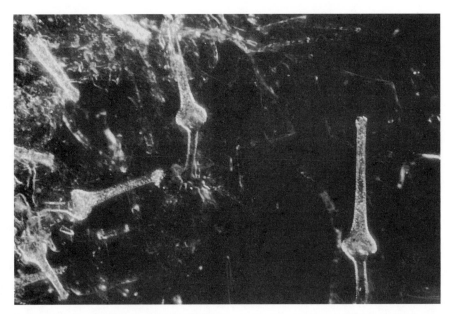

Figure 3−9. _Saksenaea vasiformis_ (CDC B-2190) after 10 days' incubation at 37°C in distilled water−yeast extract medium (magnification ×250). (From Padhye and Ajello: J Clin Microbiol 1988, with permission.)

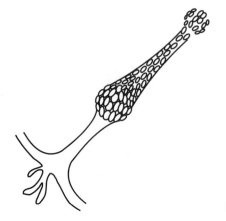

Figure 3−10. _Saksenaea_ sp.

TERMINAL VESICLE PRESENT

Sporangiophores of these organisms end in spherical vesicles from which spore-forming structures arise.

Cunninghamella Species
(Figs. 3–11 and 3–12)

Culture: On SABHI agar at room temperature, white cottony colonies grow rapidly, turning gray with age. Good growth is seen at 37°C, and some species grow at 42°C.

Microscopic: The hyphae are usually ASEPTATE. Branched SPORANGIOPHORES terminate in **VESICLES** (swollen cells) on which one-celled round SPORANGIOLA form at the tips of swollen **DENTICLES** (small toothlike projections).

Pathogenicity: Cunninghamella is a cause of zygomycosis in neutropenic patients.

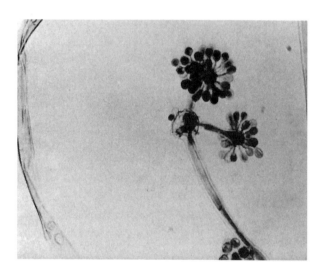

Figure 3–11. *Cunninghamella* sp. (From Koneman, et al: Practical Laboratory Mycology, ed 2. Williams & Wilkins, Baltimore, 1978, with permission.)

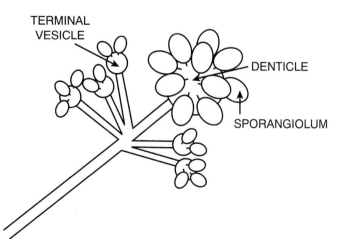

Figure 3–12. *Cunninghamella* sp.

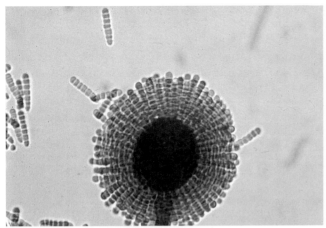

Figure 3–13. *Syncephalastrum* sp., LPCB stain (magnification ×450).

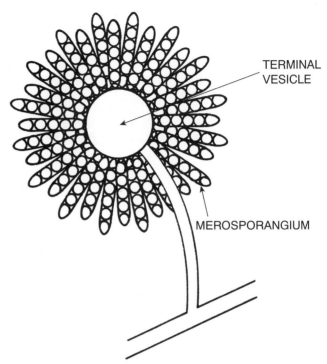

Figure 3–14. *Syncephalastrum* sp.

***Syncephalastrum*
Species**
(Figs. 3–13 and 3–14)

Culture: On SABHI agar at room temperature, a woolly dark colony rapidly matures (Color Plate 25).

Microscopic: The mycelium is usually ASEPTATE. Branched SPORANGIOPHORES terminate in vesicles. Round SPORANGIOSPORES form in a row within cylindrical **MEROSPORANGIA** (specialized sporangia) which radiate around the entire surface of the vesicle. Rudimentary rhizoids are seen. The microscopic morphology of *Syncephalastrum* sp. may easily be confused with that of *Aspergillus* sp.; however, the latter has septate hyphae, no rhizoids, and vesicles surrounded by phialides from which phialoconidia arise in chains (see Chart 3-3).

Pathogenicity: Syncephalastrum sp. is not known to be a human pathogen.

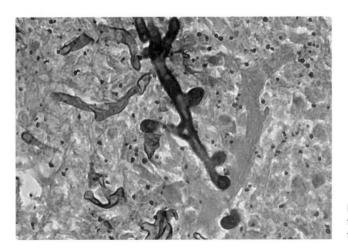

Figure 3–15. Zygomycosis, hematoxylin and eosin stain (magnification ×450).

ZYGOMYCOSIS (MUCORMYCOSIS, PHYCOMYCOSIS)

Zygomycosis (Fig. 3-15) is an acute fungus infection caused by fungi from the phylum Zygomycota. These fungi commonly grow on bread and fruits. Spores become airborne and, if the patient is in acidosis, as with uncontrolled diabetes or malnutrition, or is on corticosteroids, antibiotics, or antileukemic drugs, the spores may infect the nasal sinuses and **orbital** (eye) area. The infection rapidly spreads to adjacent blood vessels, causing necrosis and vascular **thrombosis** (blood clots). From there it spreads to the brain and meninges and produces a rapidly fatal meningoencephalitis. The disease may disseminate to the lungs and gastrointestinal tract. Death ensues two to ten days after the initial sinus/eye infection. A chronic, self-limiting form of zygomycosis has been observed in subcutaneous lesions, and a more serious form of acute progressive cellulitis of the leg was reported in diabetic patients. Direct mounts of specimens from all types of zygomycosis show branching and large ribbonlike aseptate hyphae, and round sporangia may be present. Diagnosis is confirmed with repeated isolation of the organism. Since zygomycosis of the sinuses, orbital area, and meninges is so rapidly fatal, the physician should begin treatment as soon as the disease is suspected. Treatment with amphotericin B is usually successful if initiated promptly.

STUDY QUESTIONS

1. In your own words, describe at least five common properties that fungal opportunists possess.

2. From Figure 3–16, fill in the blanks:

   A. _____
   B. _____
   C. _____

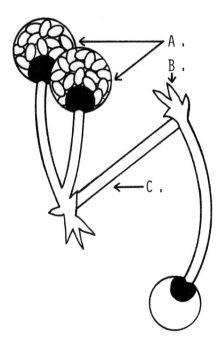

Figure 3–16. Study question demonstration.

STOP HERE UNTIL YOU HAVE COMPLETED THE QUESTIONS.

Look up the answers in the back of the book. If you missed more than two of them, go back and review the section on common properties of fungal opportunists and the section on aseptate opportunists. Correctly complete any missed study questions before proceeding further.

SEPTATE OPPORTUNISTS

Hyphae of most opportunists contain cross-walls. Those of medical importance fall into the phylum Deuteromycota. The septate opportunists may be divided into those that are **dematiaceous** (dark-colored hyphae and/or conidia), and those that are **hyaline** (light-colored hyphae and conidia) (Chart 3-2). Organisms with dark hyphae on tease mounts also have dark green to black colonies, especially on the colony reverse. The colonial color aids in the initial identification. Hyaline organisms exhibit light-colored colonial aerial hyphae, but they may be covered over with brightly colored conidia; thus, a tease mount is required. In the following descriptions, key identifying features are capitalized.

DEMATIACEOUS OPPORTUNISTS

Opportunists with dark-colored hyphae may cause **phaeohyphomycosis** (infection caused by dematiaceous fungi).

Alternaria Species
(Figs. 3–17 and 3–18)

Culture: On SABHI agar at room temperature, the light gray, woolly colony rapidly matures to dark greenish black or brown, with a black reverse (see Color Plate 16).

Microscopic: Reproductive structures and hyphae are DARK. The CHAINED PORO-CONIDIA, which contain HORIZONTAL and VERTICAL SEPTA, have club-shaped bases with tapered apices. If the poroconidia are not in chains, they may be mistaken for the opportunist *Stemphylium* (see Fig. 3–32).

Pathogenicity: *Alternaria* has been reported in keratomycosis, skin infections, osteomyelitis, pulmonary disease, and nasal septum infection.

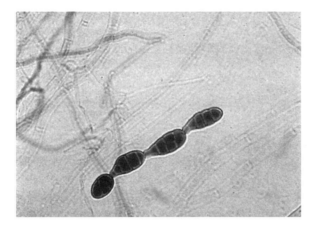

Figure 3–17. *Alternaria* sp., LPCB stain (magnification ×450).

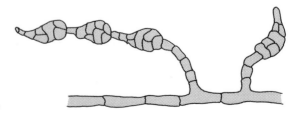

Figure 3–18. *Alternaria* sp.

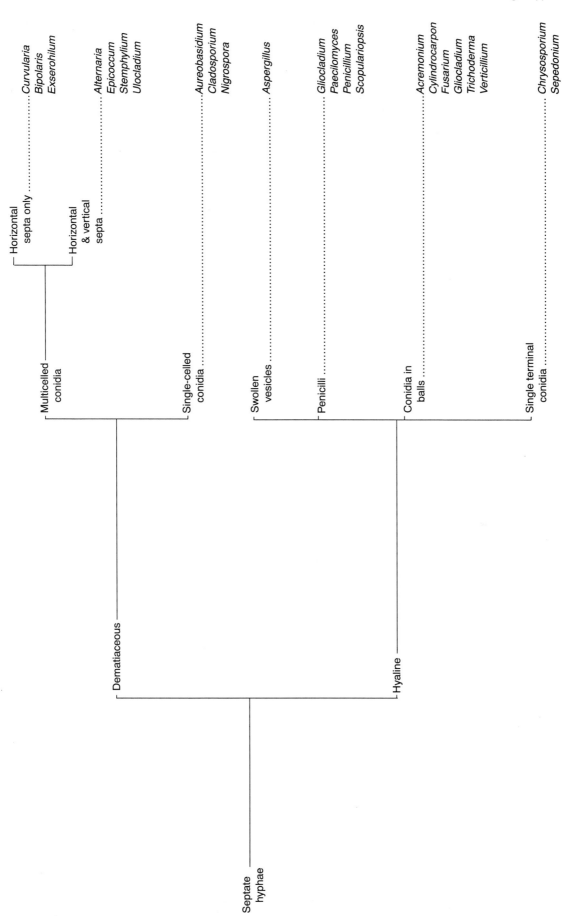

CHART 3-2. FLOW DIAGRAM FOR IDENTIFICATION OF SEPTATE FUNGAL OPPORTUNISTS*

Septate hyphae

Dematiaceous

Multicelled conidia

Horizontal septa only .... *Curvularia*
Bipolaris
Exserohilum

Horizontal & vertical septa .... *Alternaria*
Epicoccum
Stemphylium
Ulocladium

Single-celled conidia .... *Aureobasidium*
Cladosporium
Nigrospora

Hyaline

Swollen vesicles .... *Aspergillus*

Penicilli .... *Gliocladium*
Paecilomyces
Penicillium
Scopulariopsis

Conidia in balls .... *Acremonium*
Cylindrocarpon
Fusarium
Gliocladium
Trichoderma
Verticillium

Single terminal conidia .... *Chrysosporium*
Sepedonium

*Modified from Koneman, EW, et al: Practical Laboratory Mycology, ed 3. Williams & Wilkins, Baltimore, 1985.

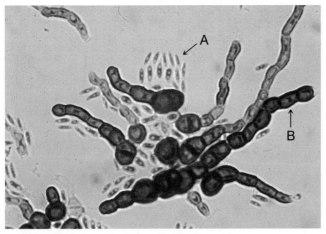

Figure 3–19. *Aureobasidium* sp., LPCB stain (magnification ×450). Arrow A indicates hyaline blastoconidia; arrow B shows dark arthroconidia.

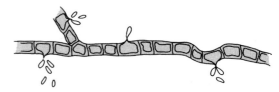

Figure 3–20. *Aureobasidium* sp.

Aureobasidium Species
(Figs. 3–19 and 3–20)

Culture: On SABHI agar at room temperature, colonies are initially shiny white and yeastlike. With age, they become shiny black and leathery with a white fringe (BLACK YEAST) (see Color Plate 17).

Microscopic: Light to DARK brown conidiophores are not differentiated from the hyphae. Short DENTICLES support HYALINE solitary or clustered CONIDIA, from which secondary blastoconidia may arise. With age, conidiophores become dark, one- to two-celled ARTHROCONIDIA.

Pathogenicity: Aureobasidium has been reported in a case of foot and leg lesions, in allergies, and in a case of cheloid blastomycosis.

Bipolaris Species
(Figs. 3–21 and 3–22)

Culture: On SABHI agar at room temperature, the rapid-growing colony is velvety or woolly, at first appearing grayish-brown; later the center is matted and black, and the reverse is light or dark (see Color Plate 20).

Microscopic: The septate hyphae are DARK. Numerous dark CYLINDRICAL, four- or five-celled POROCONIDIA with TRUNCATE **HILA** (points of attachment) are usually present in clusters along a BENT-KNEE shaped CONIDIOPHORE. When a poroconidium germinates, germ tubes may arise from one or both POLES (ends) and grow along the axis of the conidium. *Bipolaris* may be confused with the rarely pathogenic *Drechslera* sp., but the poroconidia of the latter have rounded, nonprotruding hila and germ tubes that arise perpendicular to the axis of the conidium.

Pathogenicity: Bipolaris frequently causes keratomycosis and fungal sinusitis, or occasionally subcutaneous abscesses or phaeohyphomycosis. Meningitis, allergies, and peritonitis also have been reported. Long-term therapy with amphotericin B may be effective in some, but not all, cases.

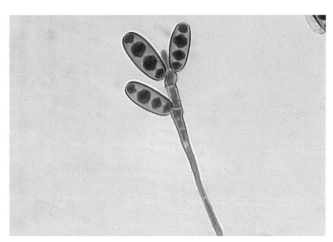

Figure 3–21. *Bipolaris* sp., LPCB stain (magnification ×450).

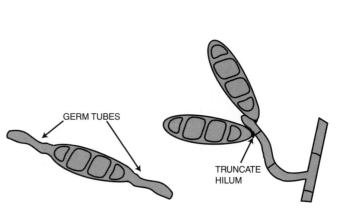

GERM TUBES

TRUNCATE HILUM

Figure 3–22. *Bipolaris* sp.

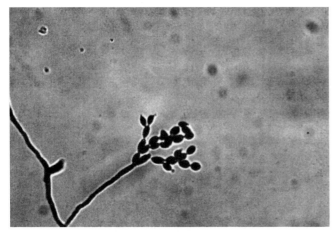

Figure 3−23. *Cladosporium* sp., LPCB stain (magnification ×450).

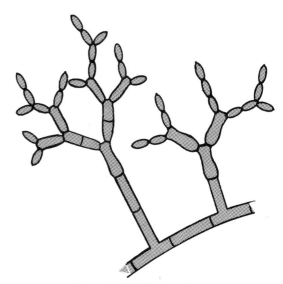

Figure 3−24. *Cladosporium* sp.

Cladosporium (Hormodendrum) Species
(Figs 3−23 and 3−24)

Culture: On SABHI agar at room temperature, the colony is moderately slow-growing for an opportunist, requiring 7 days. It is powdery or velvety, heaped and folded, and dark gray-green with the reverse black (see Color Plate 18).

Microscopic: The septate hyphae are DARK-colored. Short CHAINS of dark one- to four-celled BLASTOCONIDIA with a distinct SCAR at each point of attachment are borne from REPEATEDLY FORKING **SHIELD CELLS** (shield-shaped conidiogenous cells).

Other comments: In the past, opportunist strains of the genus were differentiated from pathogenic ones by the former's ability to hydrolyze nutrient gelatin. This test is not reliable and criteria such as growth rate, microscopic morphology, and clinical picture should be used instead.

Pathogenicity: Cladosporium may cause keratomycosis and allergies.

***Curvularia* Species**
(Figs. 3−25 and 3−26)

Culture: On SABHI agar at room temperature, the colony is moderately rapid-growing, cottony, and white, light pink, orange, or green, with a brown reverse (see Color Plate 19).

Microscopic: The septate mycelium is DARK. Large, four- to five-celled, dark POROCONIDIA are borne on a BENT-KNEE shaped CONIDIOPHORE. The poroconidia are centrally distended owing to an OVER-ENLARGED CENTRAL CELL, and the ends are lighter than the middle.

Pathogenicity: Curvularia usually causes keratomycosis, but occasionally it may produce **mycetoma** (draining subcutaneous lesions on the extremities), endocarditis, pulmonary infection, allergies, and infection of the nasal septum.

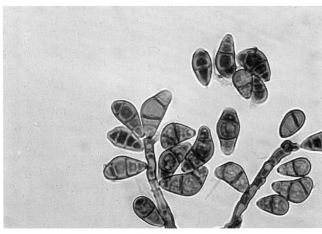

Figure 3−25. *Curvularia* sp., LPCB stain (magnification ×450).

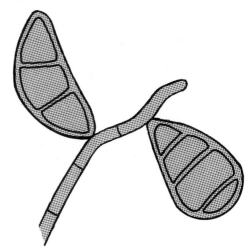

Figure 3−26. *Curvularia* sp.

Exserohilum Species
(Figs. 3−27 and 3−28)

Culture: On SABHI agar at room temperature, the colony is rapid-growing with a light grayish woolly appearance at first, which becomes dark gray to black with a black reverse.

Microscopic: The septate hyphae are DARK. Long, dark, CYLINDRICAL POROCONIDIA with 6 to 14 or more cells, and distinct, protruding, TRUNCATE HILA occur in clusters.

Exserohilum resembles the nonpathogenic *Helminthosporium* sp., but the former has a BENT-KNEE shaped CONIDIOPHORE, while the latter does not. *Exserohilum* resembles *Bipolaris* and *Drechslera,* but the former has more cells in the conidia.

Pathogenicity: Exserohilum is most often a cause of phaeohyphomycosis or fungal sinusitis, but an infected heart valve prosthesis, an aortic embolus, a corneal ulcer, and meningitis have been reported. Infections may require long-term therapy with amphotericin B.

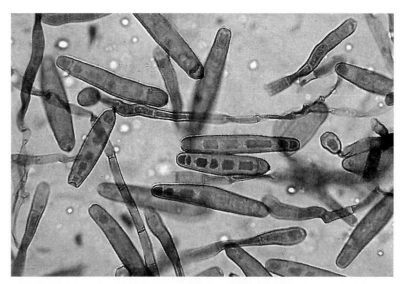

Figure 3−27. *Exserohilum* sp., LPCB stain (magnification ×500). (From Baron, et al: Bailey and Scott's Diagnostic Microbiology. Mosby-Yearbook, Inc. St. Louis, 1994, with permission.)

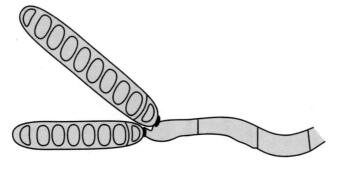

Figure 3−28. *Exserohilum* sp.

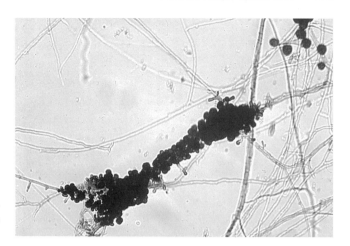

Figure 3–29. Sporodchia, *Epicoccum* sp., LPCB stain (magnification ×100).

Epicoccum Species

Culture: On SABHI agar at room temperature, colonial rings of yellow, orange, and brown are seen, and pigments of the same color may diffuse into the agar (see Color Plate 21).

Microscopic: Thick clusters of **SPORODCHIA** (short conidiophores) (Fig. 3–29) support terminal **DARK** round conidia with unconstricted **HORIZONTAL** and **VERTICAL** **SEPTA**. With age, the conidia become rough-walled. *Epicoccum* (Fig. 3–30) superficially resembles the opportunists *Ulocladium* (Fig. 3–31) and *Stemphylium*. Figure 3–32 summarizes the differences.

Pathogenicity: *Epicoccum* has been associated with allergies.

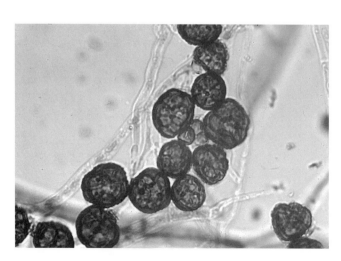

Figure 3–30. *Epicoccum* sp., LPCB stain (magnification ×450).

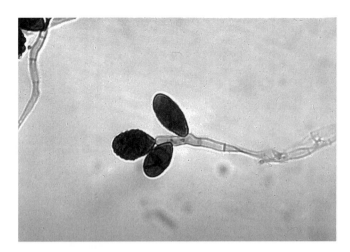

Figure 3–31. *Ulocladium* sp., LPCB stain (magnification ×450).

1. Dark round conidia	Dark round to oval poroconidia	Dark oval poroconidia
2. Unconstricted horizontal and vertical septa in conidia	Unconstricted	Constricted
3. Sporodchia	No sporodchia: bent-knee shaped conidiophore	No sporodchia: new poro-conidium produced through old scar
4. Orange colony, reverse brown	Gray to black colony, reverse black	Gray to black colony, reverse light gray

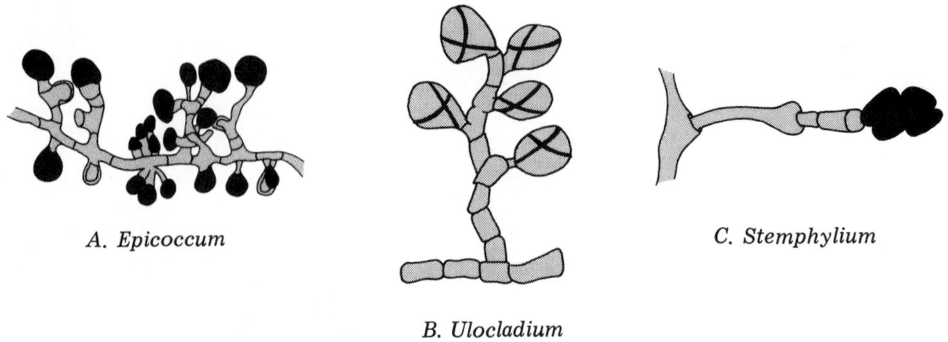

A. Epicoccum

B. Ulocladium

C. Stemphylium

Figure 3–32. Differentiation of *Epicoccum, Ulocladium,* and *Stemphylium.*

Nigrospora Species
(Figs. 3–33 and 3–34)

Culture: On SABHI agar at room temperature, a white, woolly colony with a black reverse rapidly fills the plate (see Color Plate 22). With age, the aerial mycelium turns gray.

Microscopic: The hyphae are dark. SHORT, FAT CONIDIOPHORES support SINGLE, oval, smooth-walled, BLACK CONIDIA at the tips.

Pathogenicity: Nigrospora has been reported as a causative agent of keratomycosis.

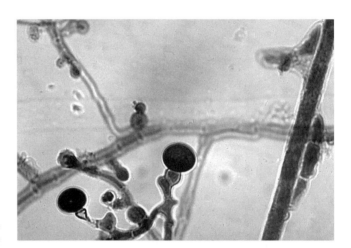

Figure 3–33. _Nigrospora_ sp., LPCB stain (magnification ×450).

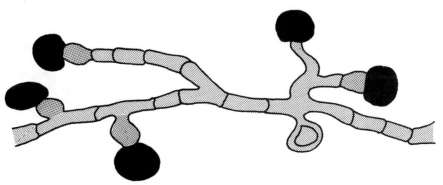

Figure 3–34. _Nigrospora_ sp.

STUDY QUESTIONS

1. Fill in the blank: If the conidia of *Alternaria* sp. are young and therefore not in chains, they may be mistaken for those of _____ .

2. Circle the correct answer(s).

   Which of the following possess conidia with vertical and horizontal cross-walls?

   A. *Curvularia* sp.

   B. *Ulocladium* sp.

   C. *Aureobasidium* sp.

   D. *Epicoccum* sp.

   E. *Bipolaris* sp.

   F. *Alternaria* sp.

   G. *Stemphylium* sp.

3. Place the letter of the answer from Column B in front of the corresponding words in Column A. An answer may be used more than once.

Column A	Column B
_____ Black yeast	A. *Nigrospora* sp
_____ Shield cells	B. *Ulocladium* sp.
_____ Enlarged central cell	C. *Aureobasidium* sp.
_____ Arthroconidia	D. *Bipolaris* sp.
_____ Single, one-celled, black conidia	E. *Cladosporium* sp.
	F. *Curvularia* sp.

STOP HERE UNTIL YOU HAVE COMPLETED THE QUESTIONS.

Look up the answers in the back of the book. If you missed more than two, go back and repeat the section on dematiaceous opportunists. Correctly complete any missed questions before proceeding.

HYALINE OPPORTUNISTS

Opportunists with light-colored hyphae may cause **hyalohyphomycosis** (infection caused by hyaline fungi).

Acremonium (Cephalosporium) Species
(Figs. 3–35 and 3–36)

Culture: On SABHI agar at room temperature, the colony is rapid-growing. It is wrinkled, membranous, and white, gray, or rose, later becoming covered with loose aerial mycelium (see Color Plate 23). The reverse is colorless, pale yellow, or pinkish.

Microscopic: The mycelium is septate. Unbranched TAPERING CONIDIOPHORES support closely packed BALLS of sickle- or elliptical-shaped CONIDIA. If the conidiophores are in whorls around the hyphae, *Acremonium* may resemble the opportunist *Verticillium;* however, *Verticillium* does not exhibit tapering conidiophores. If the conidia are more loosely packed, *Acremonium* may resemble *Sporothrix schenckii* (covered in Module 6), but *Sporothrix* forms a yeast at 37°C, while *Acremonium* does not.

Pathogenicity: Acremonium may cause keratomycosis, rarely mycetoma, lesions of hard palate, meningitis, arthritis and systemic disease.

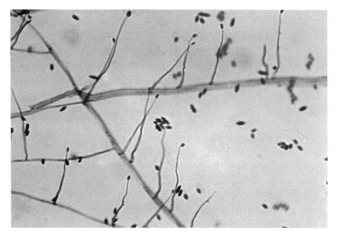

Figure 3–35. *Acremonium* sp., LPCB stain (magnification ×450).

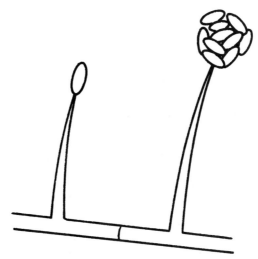

Figure 3–36. *Acremonium* sp.

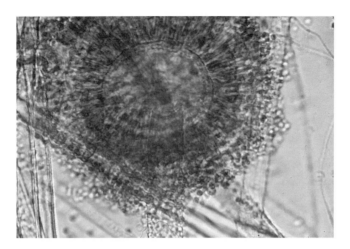

Figure 3–37. *Aspergillus* sp., LPCB stain (magnification ×450).

Aspergillus Species
(Figs. 3–37 and 3–38)

If possible, this genus should be speciated, especially *A. fumigatus* (see Chart 3-3).

Culture: On SABHI agar at room temperature, the rapid-growing colony is rugose and velvety. Various colors are due to dense production of conidia: blue, green, yellow, black, and white (see color Plates 8 and 24).

Microscopic: The mycelium is septate. Unbranched, rough or smooth conidiophores with a FOOT CELL at their base support a large VESICLE at their tip. The vesicle in turn supports short, flask-shaped PHIALIDES (old name; sterigmata) in a SINGLE or DOUBLE ROW, which produce CHAINS of smooth or rough PHIALOCONIDIA. *Aspergillus* sp. must not be confused with the similar-appearing zygomycete, *Syncephalastrum* sp. (see Figs. 3–13 and 3–14 and Color Plate 25), which is aseptate, possesses no phialides, and exhibits chains of spores in tubes (merosporangia) off the vesicle.

Other comments: **A. fumigatus** grows at 45°C, while most other *Aspergillus* species do not.

Pathogenicity: **A. fumigatus** is the most common opportunistic pathogen of the genus. It causes disseminated aspergillosis, pulmonary disease, and allergic bronchopulmonary disease (farmer's lung), as well as keratomycosis, otomycosis, and infection of the nasal sinuses.

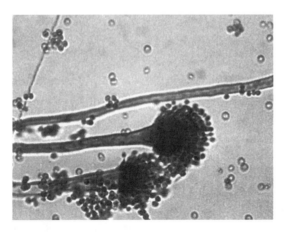

Figure 3–38. *Aspergillus fumigatus*, LPCB stain (magnification ×450).

CHART 3–3. IDENTIFICATION OF THE MOST COMMON SPECIES OF ASPERGILLUS*

	A. Fumigatus[a]	A. Niger	A. Flavus	A. Versicolor	A. Nidulans	A. Glaucus Group	A. Terreus	A. Clavatus
PATHOGENICITY	Most common cause of aspergillosis	Usually considered a contaminant, but also known to cause disease in the debilitated	Usually a contaminant but also known to cause disease; commonly associated with aflatoxins	Usually considered a contaminant, but has been known to cause disease	Usually considered a contaminant, but has been involved in infections	Commonly known as a contaminant, but also known to cause infection under certain conditions	Commonly considered a contaminant, but also known to cause infection	Commonly considered a contaminant
MACROSCOPIC MORPHOLOGY[b]	Velvety or powdery, at first white, then turning dark greenish to gray. Reverse white to tan	Woolly, at first white to yellow, then turning black. Reverse white to yellow	Velvety, yellow to green or brown Reverse goldish to red brown	Velvety; at first white, then yellow, orangey, tan, green, or occasionally pinkish. Reverse white; may be yellow, orange, or red	Velvety; usually green, but buff to yellow where cleistothecia form. Reverse purplish red becoming dark	Feltlike; green with yellow areas; occasionally brown. Reverse yellowish to maroon (grows best with 20% sucrose added to the medium)	Usually velvety, cinnamon brown. Reverse white to brown	Feltlike, blue green. Reverse white, may become brown with age
MICROSCOPIC MORPHOLOGY OF CONIDIOPHORES	Short (<300 μm) Smooth	Long Smooth	Variable length Rough, pitted, spiny	Long Smooth	Short (<250 μm) Smooth, brown	Variable length Smooth	Short (<250 μm) Smooth	Long Smooth
MICROSCOPIC MORPHOLOGY OF PHIALIDES	Uniseriate, usually only on upper two thirds of vesicle, parallel to axis of conidiophore	Biseriate, cover entire vesicle, form "radiate" head	Uniseriate and biseriate, cover entire vesicle, point out in all directions	Biseriate, loosely radiate, cover most of vesicle (Hülle cells may be present)	Biseriate, short columnar. Cleistothecia usually present with reddish ascospores; Hülle cells often abundant.	Uniseriate, radiate to very loosely columnar, cover entire vesicle (cleistothecia generally present)	Biseriate, compactly columnar (round hyaline cells produced on mycelium submerged in agar)	Uniseriate, closely crowded on huge clavate vesicle (approximately 200 × 40 μm)

*From Larone, DH: Medically Important Fungi: A Guide to Identification, ed 3. ASM Press, Washington, DC, 1995.

[a]A. fumigatus grows well at 45°C or higher.

[b]Classically studied on Czapek-Dox agar; on Sabouraud dextrose agar, most species of Aspergillus grown luxuriantly but not always characteristically.

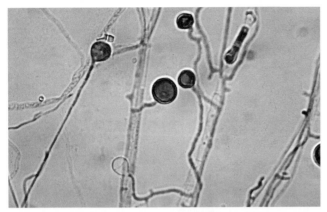

Figure 3–39. *Chrysosporium* sp., LPCB stain (magnification ×450).

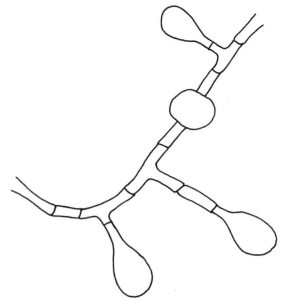

Figure 3–40. *Chrysosporium* sp.

***Chrysosporium*
Species**
(Figs. 3–39 and 3–40)

Culture: On SABHI agar at room temperature, a heaped, velvety, buff-colored colony rapidly forms, with a white, yellow, or reddish brown reverse (see Color Plate 26).

Microscopic: SINGLE, round to club-shaped, smooth or rough CONIDIA perch on top of short conidiophores, which are poorly differentiated from the vegetative mycelium. Conidia also develop directly off the hyphae, and swollen arthroconidia may be present. *Chrysosporium* colonially and microscopically resembles the subcutaneous pathogen *Scedosporium apiospermum* (see Module 6) and the mold phase of the systemic dimorphs *Blastomyces dermatitidis* and *Histoplasma capsulatum* (see Module 7). However, *Chrysosporium* is a rapid grower, while *Scedosporium* is intermediate and *Blastomyces* and *Histoplasma* are slow. Unlike the dimorphs, *Chrysosporium* cannot be converted to a yeast phase at 37°C. *Scedosporium* also does not form a yeast phase but can be separated on the basis of clinical manifestations, annellides, and by the common presence of sexual stage cleistothecia.

Pathogenicity: Chrysosporium has rarely been reported as a pathogen.

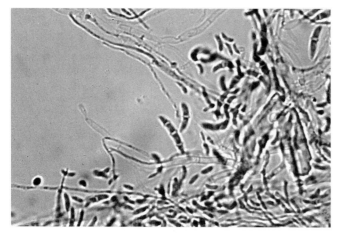

Figure 3–41. *Fusarium* sp., LPCB stain (magnification ×450).

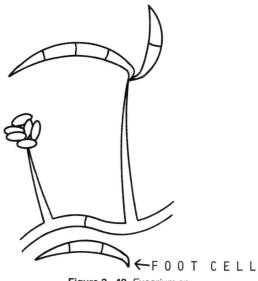

Figure 3–42. *Fusarium* sp.

Fusarium Species
(Figs. 3–41 and 3–42)

Culture: On SABHI agar at room temperature, the rapid-growing colony is white at first and woolly or cottony. Later it becomes LAVENDER, or sometimes yellow or orange, with a light reverse (see Color Plate 27).

Microscopic: The mycelium is septate. Conidiophores are single or branching, occasionally producing whorls, and they terminate in tapering phialides. Microphialoconidia are one-celled and occur in balls; if macrophialoconidia are not exhibited, *Fusarium* may be mistaken for *Acremonium*. Diagnostic MACROPHIALOCONIDIA are two- to five-celled, BANANA- or CYLINDRICAL-SHAPED, with a distinctive FOOT CELL at the point of attachment. The opportunist *Cylindrocarpon* produces similar-appearing macrophialoconidia; however, the ends are rounded, there are no foot cells, and one to ten septa may occur. Chlamydoconidia are common in *Fusarium*.

Pathogenicity: Fusarium is the most common cause of keratomycosis. It has also been isolated from skin lesions on burn patients, in **onychomycosis** (nail infection), otomycosis, varicose ulcers, mycetoma, osteomyelitis following trauma, and disseminated infection.

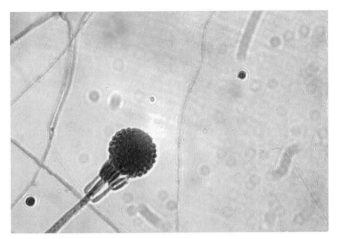

Figure 3–43. *Gliocladium* sp., LPCB stain (magnification ×450).

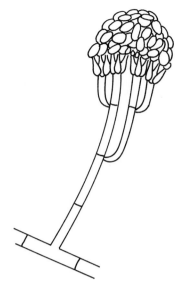

Figure 3–44. *Gliocladium* sp.

Gliocladium Species
(Figs. 3–43 and 3–44)

Culture: On SABHI agar at room temperature, the colony is initially white but rapidly fills the plate with a green, furry growth mimicking a GREEN LAWN (see Color Plate 28). Some strains may remain white or turn rose colored. The reverse is white. The opportunist *Trichoderma* is also initially white and later green; however, the color is usually more yellowish green, and the growth is cottony.

Microscopic: **PENICILLI** (singular, penicillus) (brushlike conidiophores) bear flask-shaped PHIALIDES, which in turn produce terminal masses of hyaline to green PHIALOCONIDIA, held together in a LARGE BALL by a gelatinous matrix. Young penicilli with only one or two branches may be mistaken for *Trichoderma* and *Verticillium*, which exhibit single or whorled phialides with terminal balls of phialoconidia. *Trichoderma* structures are smaller and more delicate than *Gliocladium*; also, with careful searching, no penicilli should be found with either *Trichoderma* or *Verticillium*.

Pathogenicity: Gliocladium is not known to be a human pathogen.

Paecilomyces Species
(Figs. 3–45 and 3–46)

Culture: On SABHI agar at room temperature, the powdery, velvety, or cottony mycelium very rapidly matures to an OLIVE TAN (see Color Plate 29), although shades of violet or brown may be seen.

Microscopic: Single, whorled, or penicillus-type ELONGATED PHIALIDES bear CHAINS of smooth or rough, hyaline to pigmented oval CONIDIA. Microscopically, *Paecilomyces* maintains a close semblance to the opportunists *Penicillium* and *Verticillium*, but the latter fungi do not exhibit elongated phialides.

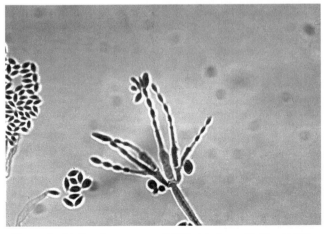

Figure 3–45. *Paecilomyces* sp., LPCB stain (magnification ×450).

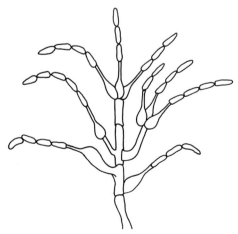

Figure 3–46. *Paecilomyces* sp.

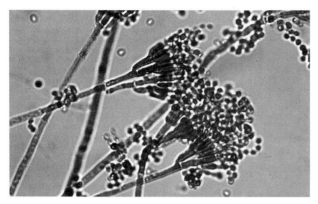

Figure 3–47. *Penicillium* sp., LPCB stain (magnification ×450).

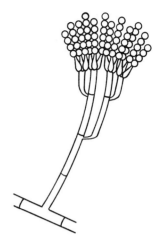

Figure 3–48. *Penicillium* sp.

Pathogenicity: Paecilomyces has been implicated in cases of penicilliosis, endophthalmitis, endocarditis, pleural effusion, and skin lesions.

***Penicillium* Species**
(Figs. 3–47 to 3–49)

Culture: On SABHI agar at room temperature, the rapid-growing colony is initially velvety and white, later becoming powdery and BLUE GREEN with a white periphery and colorless reverse (see Color Plate 30).

Microscopic: The mycelium is septate. PENICILLI bear flask-shaped PHIALIDES, which in turn support CHAINS of round PHIALOCONIDIA. Conidiophores and phialoconidia may be hyaline to pigmented, and smooth to rough, depending on species.

Pathogenicity: Penicillium causes keratomycosis, penicilliosis, otomycosis, onychomycosis, and rarely, deep infection.

Penicillium marneffei (Fig. 3–49)
Culture: On SABHI agar at room temperature, the rapid-growing, grayish floccose colonies have a finely wrinkled surface and a DARK RED pigment that diffuses throughout the agar. At 37°C, on blood agar, yeastlike colonies may appear in 3 to 4 days and are grayish white, waxy and attached to the agar surface.

Microscopic: At room temperature, the septate mycelium is typical of *Penicillium* with conidiophores bearing up to five short broad **METULAE** (branched conidiophores). The WIDE PHIALIDES, which taper to narrow apices, are borne in groups of four to six on the metulae. Smooth, lemon-shaped PHIALOCONIDIA occur in chains. Growth at 37°C on blood agar is yeastlike; filamentous forms and yeast forms may be seen.

Pathogenicity: Penicillium marneffei causes a disseminated form of penicilliosis.

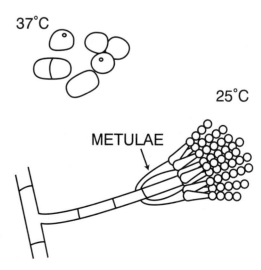

Figure 3–49. Mold and yeast phases, *Penicillium marneffei.*

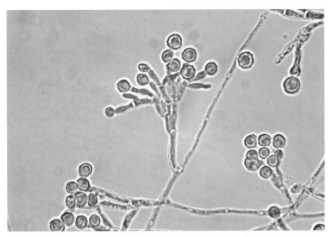

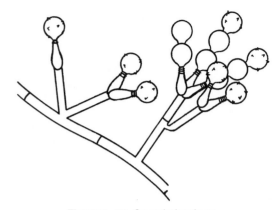

Figure 3–51. *Scopulariopsis* sp.

Figure 3–50. *Scopulariopsis* sp., LPCB stain (magnification ×450).

Scopulariopsis Species
(Figs. 3–50 and 3–51)

Culture: On SABHI agar at room temperature, the rapid-growing colony is velvety, rugose, and white, later becoming light tan or brown, with a tan reverse (see Color Plate 31).

Microscopic: The mycelium is septate. Single, unbranching, or PENICILLUS-type ANNELLOPHORES bear flask-shaped ANNELLIDES, which in turn support large LEMON-SHAPED ANNELLOCONIDIA in chains. With age, the conidia become **echinulate,** or SPINY.

Pathogenicity: Scopulariopsis causes keratomycosis, rarely bronchopulmonary disease (penicilliosis), otomycosis, and onychomycosis. It has been reported in an infection of the ankle and as the cause of an inguinal ulcer.

Sepedonium Species
(Figs. 3–52 and 3–53)

Culture: On SABHI agar at room temperature, the waxy and white colony rapidly becomes velvety and lemon-colored with a peripheral fringe, and white reverse (see Color Plate 32).

Microscopic: SINGLE or clustered, THICK-WALLED, SMOOTH TO ROUGH (MACRO) CONIDIA form at the ends of simple or branched conidiophores which are not well differentiated from the vegetative mycelium. Formerly, it was thought that single, smooth, and thin-walled, elliptical (micro)conidia were also produced: it is now thought that these only represent young macroconidia. *Sepedonium* greatly imitates the systemic dimorph *Histoplasma capsulatum* (see Module 7) which possesses macro- and microconidia, but the former does not convert to a yeast phase at 37°C.

Pathogenicity: Sepedonium is not known to be a human pathogen.

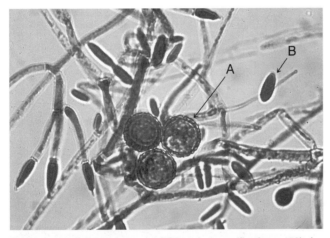

Figure 3–52. *Sepedonium* sp., LPCB stain (magnification ×450). Arrow A indicates a macroconidium; arrow B shows a previously named microconidium, now considered to be a young macroconidium.

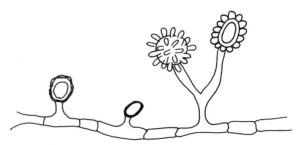

Figure 3–53. *Sepedonium* sp.

STUDY QUESTIONS

1. *Penicillium, Gliocladium, Paecilomyces,* and *Scopulariopsis* all possess a penicillus. Describe three ways in which they may be distinguished from each other.

2. *Aspergillus* and *Syncephalastrum* resemble each other microscopically. Put an A in front of each characteristic that pertains to *Aspergillus* sp., a B in front of those items that apply to *Syncephalastrum* sp., and a C where neither fungus is characterized.

_____ Aseptate

_____ Vesicles

_____ Blastoconidia

_____ Merosporangia

_____ Foot cells

_____ Phialides

A. *Aspergillus*

B. *Syncephalastrum*

C. Neither fungus

3. Circle true or false:

T   F   *Acremonium* exhibits repeatedly forking conidiophores with terminal balls of conidia.

4. The fungi listed in Column A below all possess single, one-celled, terminal conidia. The items in Column B may be used to differentiate them. Place the letter of the characteristic from Column B in front of the corresponding organism in Column A. More than one characteristic may be placed in front of each fungus.

Column A

_____ *Chrysosporium* sp.

_____ *Sepedonium* sp.

_____ *Scedosporium apiospermum*

_____ *Blastomyces dermatitidis*

_____ *Histoplasma capsulatum*

Column B

A. Dimorphic

B. Rapid growing

C. May possess microconidia

D. Cleistothecia common

E. Annellidic

STOP HERE UNTIL YOU HAVE COMPLETED THE QUESTIONS.

Look up the answers in the back of the book. If you missed more than two, go back and repeat the section on hyaline opportunists. Correctly complete any missed questions before proceeding.

OPPORTUNISTIC MYCOSES

See Chart 3-4.

Aspergillosis

Aspergillosis is usually acquired by inhalation of the conidia. It begins as a pulmonary disease, producing **granulomatous** (tumorous) lesions in the lungs or bronchi. These may be spread from the lung tissue into the surrounding blood vessels. Subsequently, the disease disseminates to the rest of the body, including the brain, gastrointestinal tract, and kidneys. This invasive pulmonary form of aspergillosis is being increasingly observed in debilitated patients receiving antibiotic, immunosuppressive, or cancer therapy. The disseminated disease is usually acute and fatal. In two characteristic forms of aspergillosis—otomycosis (external ear infection) and fungus ball (abscess)—there is no tissue invasion. Asthma attacks can be initiated in sensitized individuals by inhalation of *Aspergillus* conidia (allergic bronchopulmonary disease). Miscellaneous types of aspergillosis include myocarditis, meningitis, osteomyelitis, mycetoma, burn infection, invasion of the nasal sinuses, onychomycosis, keratomycosis, and toxin ingestion from eating contaminated foods.

CHART 3–4. SOME ORGANISMS THAT CAUSE OPPORTUNISTIC MYCOSES

Aspergillosis	Penicilliosis	Keratomycosis	Otomycosis	Sinusitis	Zygomycosis
Aspergillus flavus	Paecilomyces sp.	Absidia sp.	Aspergillus fumigatus	Aspergillus sp.	Absidia sp.
Aspergillus fumigatus	Penicillium sp.	Acremonium sp.	Aspergillus niger	Alternaria sp.	Apophysomyces sp.
Aspergillus niger	Penicillium marneffei	Actinomyces bovis	Aspergillus terreus	Bipolaris sp.	Cunninghamella sp.
Aspergillus terreus	Scopulariopsis sp.	Alternaria sp.	Candida albicans	Cladosporium sp.	Mortierella sp.
		Aspergillus flavus	Candida tropicalis	Curvularia sp.	Mucor sp.
		Aspergillus fumigatus	Epidermophyton floccosum	Exserohilum sp.	Rhizopus sp.
		Aspergillus niger	Fusarium sp.		Rhizomucor sp.
		Bipolaris sp.	Mucor sp.		Saksenaea sp.
		Candida sp.	Penicillium sp.		
		Cladosporium sp.	Rhizopus sp.		
		Curvularia sp.	Scopulariopsis sp.		
		Cylindrocarpon sp.	Trichophyton violaceum		
		Exophiala jeanselmei			
		Fusarium sp.			
		Graphium sp.			
		Mucor sp.			
		Nigrospora sp.			
		Nocardia sp.			
		Penicillium sp.			
		Phialophora verrucosa			
		Rhizopus sp.			
		Rhodotorula sp.			
		Scedosporium sp.			
		Scopulariopsis sp.			
		Sporothrix schenckii			
		Trichosporon sp.			
		Ustilago sp.			
		Volutella sp.			

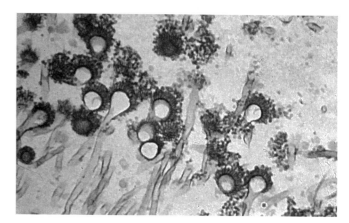

Figure 3–54. Aspergillosis, fruiting heads, Gridley's modification of periodic acid–Schiff (PAS) stain. (From Dolan, et al: Atlas of Clinical Mycology. ASCP, Washington, DC, 1975, with permission.)

Direct mounts of specimens reveal septate hyphae that branch dichotomously (Y-shaped branching) (see Color Plate 33). Specimens from fungus balls may also show the typical *Aspergillus* fruiting heads (Fig. 3–54). Classically, diagnosis is confirmed if repeated cultures of infected material grow large numbers of *Aspergillus* species. However, in cases of invasive pulmonary aspergillosis, only 25% of patients may produce positive cultures, and only half of those may possess more than one positive result. Therefore, isolation of *A. fumigatus* or *A. flavus* should not be automatically considered as laboratory contamination but rather should be judged in light of the patient's medical history. *A. fumigatus* is most commonly isolated from invasive pulmonary aspergillosis, fungus ball, and allergic bronchopulmonary disease. *A. flavus* is seen in invasive pulmonary aspergillosis and allergic bronchopulmonary disease, while *A. niger* produces fungus ball and otomycosis. Aspergillosis usually responds to treatment with amphotericin B.

Penicilliosis

Penicilliosis (or hyalohyphomycosis caused by penicillus-producing fungi) is usually acquired by inhaling the conidia of the opportunists *Penicillium, Scopulariopsis,* or *Paecilomyces.* It starts as a pulmonary disease but may spread into the adjacent blood vessels. Subsequently it disseminates to the rest of the body, including the spinal fluid, kidneys (*Penicillium*), and endocardium (*Paecilomyces, Penicillium*). Such total invasion occurs in debilitated patients. Penicilliosis may also include infections of the nails (*Scopulariopsis*), otomycosis (*Penicillium*), keratomycosis (*Penicillium, Scopulariopsis*), inguinal ulcers (*Scopulariopsis*), and allergic bronchial asthma in sensitized people (*Penicillium, Scopulariopsis*). Observing hyphae and conidia in direct mounts is in itself not significant unless the organism is also repeatedly isolated in large numbers.

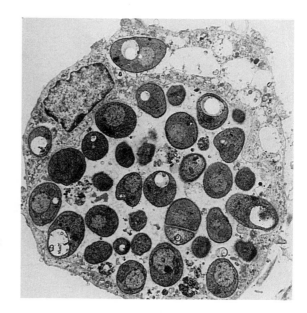

Figure 3–55. Macrophage filled with yeast bodies of *Penicillium marneffei*, uranyl acetate and lead citrate negative stain. (From Peto, et al: J Infection 1988, with permission.)

The disseminated form of penicilliosis caused by *Penicillium marneffei* is characterized by an acute onset of fever, chills, cough, weakness, loss of weight, leukocytosis, anemia and enlarged lymph nodes, spleen, and liver. It is hypothesized that the primary infection may be either pulmonary, through inhalation of the organism, or intestinal, through ingestion of the organism. The disease occurs in Southeast Asia, especially southern China, Thailand, Hong Kong, and Vietnam. Although the disease has occurred in immunocompetent individuals, it occurs most often in immunocompromised and AIDS patients, some of whom may be diagnosed in the United States or Europe following travel to Southeast Asia. Hematoxylin and eosin (H&E) stains of affected tissue reveal yeast bodies occurring intracellularly within macrophages (Fig. 3–55). These resemble the appearance of *H. capsulatum* but *Histoplasma* appears pseudoencapsulated. The yeast bodies of *P. marneffei* divide by elongating into sausage forms, developing a septum across the width of the cell, and splitting at the septum into two cells. If not treated with antifungal agents such as amphotericin B, ketoconazole, fluconazole or 5-fluorocytosine, the disseminated disease is usually fatal.

Keratomycosis

The cornea of the eye is resistant to infection. However, with predisposing factors, fungi can invade the cornea and cause keratomycosis (Fig. 3–56). The factors include trauma to the eye, use of corticosteroids (antiinflammatory medications used in conjunction with antibiotics for supposed bacterial infection of the eye), and glaucoma. A white or cream-colored infiltrate develops after the conidia germinate, and hyphal growth forms in the area of trauma. Ulceration occurs in the cornea, eventually causing scarring and subsequent blindness. Fungal lesions range from the extremely painful to the unnoticed—unnoticed possibly because of decreased sensation of the eye which follows nerve damage or long-continued wearing of contact lenses. The lesions may elicit an **inflammatory** (pus cell) response as described above, or none at all. Corneal scrapings should be taken for direct mounts and culture. Since the causative organisms are mostly opportunists, a fungus must be repeatedly isolated to be considered etiologically significant. There are over 80 fungi that may cause keratomycosis (see Chart 3-4).

The drug of choice for keratomycosis is natamycin, a polyene antifungal agent which, because of its wide spectrum of activity, is effective against yeasts as well as hyaline and dematiaceous molds. This agent is administered in the form of a 5% suspension which must be applied to the affected eye as often as every hour for the first few days. Rapid improvement of the infection usually occurs with this regimen.

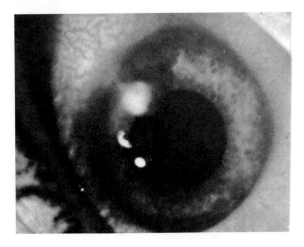

Figure 3–56. Keratomycosis. (From Beneke and Rogers: Medical Mycology Manual. Burgess, Minneapolis, 1970, with permission.)

Otomycosis   Otomycosis (Fig. 3–57) is a fungal infection of the external auditory opening or ear canal, with symptoms of inflammation, itching, scaling, and partial deafness due to the ear canal being filled with a hyphal plug. Trauma often starts the disease; the habit of cleaning the ears with matches or similar objects causes abrasions that become readily infected. Fungal infection may be secondary to a bacterial ear infection or to previous use of antibiotics. Too much heat and moisture may predispose the patient to otomycosis. Scrapings and purulent discharge are the specimens of choice for direct mount and culture. Many of the fungal etiologic agents are opportunists and thus must be repeatedly isolated in large numbers before being considered significant. Also, other organisms, such as yeasts or dermatophytes, may cause otomycosis.

Sinusitis   Sinusitis is an infection of the nasal sinuses with symptoms of sinus pain, nasal discharge, nasal obstruction, and inflammation. The syndrome may be caused by a number of bacterial or fungal species, and can be either acute or chronic. *Aspergillus* was considered the usual cause of fungal sinusitis, but in recent years, species of dematiaceous fungi such as *Bipolaris, Curvularia,* and *Alternaria* were reported most often as important agents of fungal sinusitis. It usually occurs in immunocompetent patients with a history of allergy and nasal polyps. Eosinophilia is common. Patients present with thick nasal discharge that may occasionally be bloody and contain pieces of brownish tissue. Surgical debridement is usually necessary for effective treatment of chronic sinusitis. If untreated, the paranasal sinuses, orbital sinuses or central nervous system may become involved with potentially life-threatening consequences.

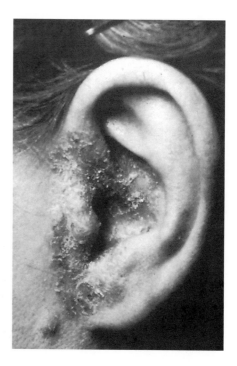

Figure 3–57. Otomycosis. (From Conant, et al: Manual of Clinical Mycology. WB Saunders, Philadelphia, 1971, with permission.)

FINAL EXAM

1. Circle the correct answer:
   Banana-shaped macrophialoconidia with foot cells are diagnostic of:

   A. *Cylindrocarpon* sp.

   B. *Nigrospora* sp.

   C. *Curvularia* sp.

   D. *Fusarium* sp.

   E. *Paecilomyces* sp.

2. Circle true or false:
   T   F   Dematiaceous organisms exhibit light-colored hyphae and/or conidia.

3. In front of numbers 1 to 3, write the letter(s) of the fungus that represents each characteristic:

   A. *Absidia* sp.   _____ 1. Produces rhizoids

   B. *Mucor* sp.   _____ 2. Branching sporangiophores

   C. *Rhizopus* sp.   _____ 3. Internodal sporangiophores

4. *Epicoccum* sp., *Ulocladium* sp., and *Stemphylium* sp. all demonstrate similar conidia. Describe at least two ways to differentiate them.

5. Circle true of false:
   T   F   Isolates of *Helminthosporium* are distinguished from *Bipolaris* in that *Helminthosporium* possess conidiophores that grow in a bent-knee fashion, while *Bipolaris* conidiophores grow straight.

6. Circle true of false:
   T   F   *Aspergillus fumigatus* produces phialides and phialoconidia only at the end of the vesicle.

7. In these blanks, write the genus identified from each drawing in the right-hand column.

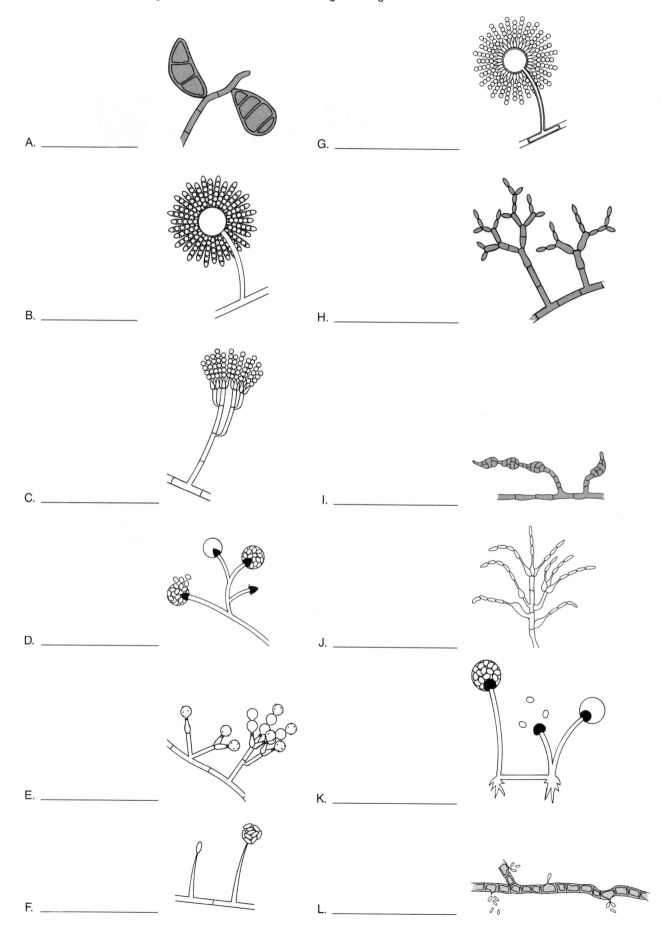

A. _____

B. _____

C. _____

D. _____

E. _____

F. _____

G. _____

H. _____

I. _____

J. _____

K. _____

L. _____

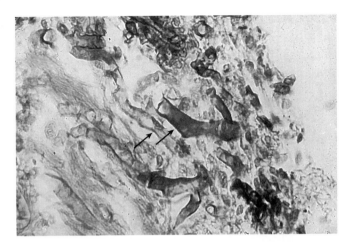

Figure 3–58. Case study demonstration, methenamine silver stain (magnification ×450). Arrows indicate hyphae.

8. Circle true or false:

T F In aspergillosis, the etiologic fungus may be isolated only once and still be considered significant.

9. Circle the letter of the correct answer(s).

Otomycosis involves:

A. external ear infections.

B. deep inner ear infections.

10. Circle true of false:

T F The cornea of the eye is easily susceptible to infection.

For questions 11 through 14, refer to the following case study and Figure 3–58.

A 10-year-old boy was admitted to the hospital in diabetic ketoacidosis. Three days later, he complained of nasal sinus blockage. Stained histologic preparations of material removed from his sinuses showed the wide, ribbonlike hyphae seen in Figure 3–58. On SABHI agar, a white cottony mold rapidly grew.

11. Which disease do you suspect, and why?

12. Circle the letter of the correct answer. Three agents of this mycosis are:

A. *Rhizomucor, Fusarium,* and *Acremonium.*

B. *Penicillium, Scopulariopsis,* and *Paecilomyces.*

C. *Absidia, Mucor,* and *Rhizopus.*

D. *Aspergillus fumigatus, Aspergillus niger,* and *Aspergillus flavus.*

E. *Cladosporium, Alternaria,* and *Bipolaris.*

13. Slide cultures of the mold revealed unbranching sporangiophores at rhizoid nodes.

Fill in the blank: The causative organism is _____.

14. Since this is an opportunistic infection, should the physician wait for repeated cultures before initiating treatment? Why or why not?

STOP HERE UNTIL YOU HAVE COMPLETED THE QUESTIONS.

Look up the answers in the back of the book. If you missed more than three, go back and repeat this module. Correctly complete any missed questions.

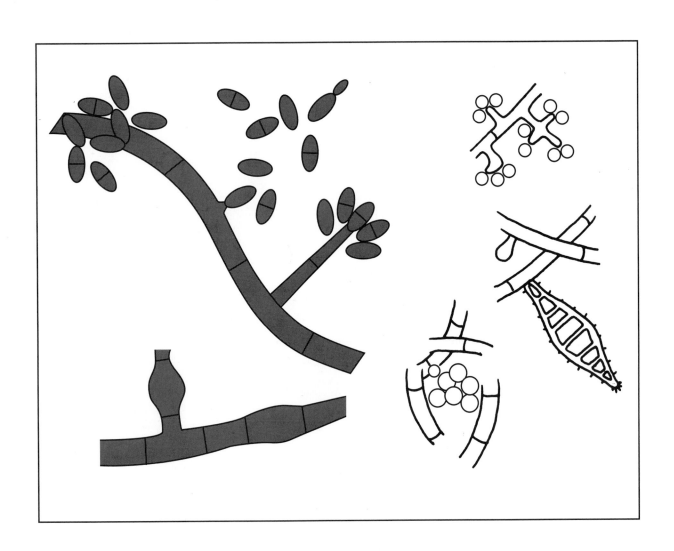

Superficial and Dermatophytic Fungi

PREREQUISITES

The learner must possess a good background knowledge in clinical microbiology and must have finished Module 1, Basics of Mycology, and Module 2, Laboratory Procedures for Fungal Culture and Isolation.

BEHAVIORAL OBJECTIVES

Upon completion of this module, the learner should be able to:

1 Compare and contrast:
   Superficial and cutaneous mycoses
   Cutaneous mycoses and dermatophytoses

2 Identify hairs with endothrix invasion, ectothrix invasion, and in vitro perforation.

3 Identify the following fungi from culture, microscopic appearance, biochemical characteristics, and mycosis produced:

   Malassezia furfur   *Epidermophyton floccosum*
   Exophiala werneckii   *Trichophyton mentagrophytes*
   Piedraia hortai   *Trichophyton rubrum*
   Trichosporon beigelii   *Trichophyton verrucosum*
   Microsporum audouinii   *Trichophyton tonsurans*
   Microsporum canis   *Trichophyton schoenleinii*
   Microsporum gypseum   *Trichophyton violaceum*

4 Briefly describe the clinical characteristics and treatment of the following mycoses and state with which organism (listed in objective 3) each is associated. State common mycosis names where appropriate.

   Pityriasis versicolor   Dermatophytosis of the body (tinea
   Tinea nigra   corporis)
   Black piedra   Dermatophytosis of the groin (tinea
   White piedra   cruris)
   Dermatophytosis of the scalp (tinea capitis) Dermatophytosis of the foot (tinea pedis)
   Dermatophytosis of the beard (tinea   Dermatophytosis of the nail (tinea
      barbae)   unguium)

5 Concerning the three dermatophyte genera:
   A. List them.
   B. State which body sites (skin, nails, ectothrix hair, endothrix hair) are infected by each genus.
   C. Describe the microscopic characteristics, especially macro- and microconidia, that are typical for each genus.

6 Discuss how the location of dermatophytosis (tinea), hair fluorescence, and growth rate aid in speciation of dermatophytes.

7 Describe the usefulness of the following in dermatophyte species identification.
Color on potato dextrose or corn meal agar
In vitro perforation of autoclaved hair
Trichophyton agars
Christenson's urea agar
Polished rice grains

Include which organisms are differentiated, how to set up each procedure, and positive and negative results.

8 Outline the chronology of a typical dermatophyte infection, and describe the area of the lesion from which positive cultures can be expected.

CONTENT OUTLINE

I. Introduction
II. Superficial organisms
  A. *Exophiala werneckii*
  B. *Malassezia furfur*
  C. *Piedraia hortai*
  D. *Trichosporon beigelii*
  E. Study questions
III. Dermatophytes
  A. General differential characteristics
    1. Location of the dermatophytosis (tinea)
    2. Hair fluorescence
    3. Growth rate
    4. Microscopic characteristics of each dermatophyte genus
    5. Physiologic tests
    6. Study questions
  B. Dermatophytes pathogenic to humans

    1. *Microsporum* species
      a. *Microsporum audouinii*
      b. *Microsporum canis*
      c. *Microsporum gypseum*
    2. *Epidermophyton* species
      a. *Epidermophyton floccosum*
    3. *Trichophyton* species
      a. Ectothrix hair invasion
        (1) *Trichophyton mentagrophytes*
        (2) *Trichophyton rubrum*
        (3) *Trichophyton verrucosum*
      b. Study questions
      c. Endothrix hair invasion
        (1) *Trichophyton schoenleinii*
        (2) *Trichophyton tonsurans*
        (3) *Trichophyton violaceum*
IV. Dermatophytosis
V. Final exam

FOLLOW-UP ACTIVITIES

1 Students may observe colonies and slide culture preparations of fungi that cause superficial and dermatophytic infections.

2 Students may be assigned unknown dermatophytes for which they must perform differential identification tests.

REFERENCES

Chong, KC, et al: Morphology of *Piedraia hortai*. Sabouraudia 9:157, 1975.

Gregurek-Novak, T, et al: Defective phagocytosis in chronic trichophytosis. J Med Vet Mycol 31:115, 1993.

Faergemann, J, et al: *Trichophyton rubrum* abscesses in immunocompromised patients: a case report. Acta Derm Venereol 69:244, 1989.

Fusaro, M, et al: Tinea pedis caused by *Trichophyton violaceum*. Am J Clin Pathol 80:110, 1983.

Hageage, GJ and Harrington, BJ: Use of calcofluor white in clinical mycology. Lab Med 15:109, 1984.

Kane, J and Smitka, C: Early detection and identification of *Trichophyton verrucosum*. J Clin Microbiol 8:740, 1978.

King, D, et al: Primary invasive cutaneous *Microsporum canis* infections in immunocompromised patients. J Clin Microbiol 34:460, 1996.

Koneman, EW, et al: Practical Laboratory Mycology, ed 3. Williams & Wilkins, Baltimore, 1985.

Knudsen, EA: Experimental dermatophyte infection: The extent of the fungal invasion. Acta Derm Venereol 69:247, 1989.

Kwon-Chung, KJ and Bennett, JE: Medical Mycology, Lea & Febiger, Philadelphia, 1992.

Larone, DH: Medically Important Fungi, ed 3. ASM Press, Washington, DC, 1995.

Lestringant, GG, et al: Deep dermatophytosis of *Trichophyton rubrum* and *T. verrucosum* in an immunosuppressed patient. Int J Dermatol 27:707, 1988.

Mok, WY: Nature and identification of *Exophiala werneckii*. J Clin Microbiol 16:976, 1982.

Naka, W, et al: Application of neutral red staining for evaluation of the viability of dermatophytes and *Candida* in human skin scales. J Med Vet Mycol 32:101, 1994.

Nelson, SC, et al: Improved detection of *Malassezia* species in lipid-supplemented Peds Plus blood cultures bottles. J Clin Microbiol 33:1005, 1995.

Novick, NL, et al: Invasive *Trichophyton rubrum* infection in an immunocompromised host. Am J Med 82:321, 1987.

Odds, FC, et al: Nomenclature of fungal diseases: a report and recommendations from a subcommittee of the International Society for Human and Animal Mycology (ISHAM). J Med Vet Mycol 30:1, 1992.

Philpot, CM: The use of nutritional tests for the differentiation of dermatophytes. Sabouraudia 15:141, 1977.

Rezusta, A, et al: Differentiation between *Trichophyton mentagrophytes* and *Trichophyton rubrum* by sorbitol assimilation. J Clin Microbiol 29:219, 1991.

Richet, HM, et al: Cluster of *Malassezia furfur* pulmonary infections in infants in a neonatal intensive-care unit. J Clin Microbiol 27:1197, 1989.

Samdani, AJ, et al: The effect of dermatophyte species and density of infection on the pathology of ringworm. J Med Vet Mycol 29:279, 1991.

Shadomy, HJ and Philpot, CM: Utilization of standard laboratory methods in the laboratory diagnosis of problem dermatophytes. Am J Clin Pathol 74:197, 1980.

Tanaka, S, et al: Advances in dermatophytes and dermatophytosis. J Med Vet Mycol 30(Suppl 1):29, 1992.

Teglia, O, et al: *Malassezia furfur* infections. Infect Control Hosp Epidemiol 12:676, 1991.

Vargo, K and Cohen, BA: Prevalence of undetected tinea capitis in household members of children with disease. Pediatrics 92:155, 1993.

Walsh, T, et al: *Trichosporon beigelii,* an emerging pathogen resistant to amphotericin B. J Clin Microbiol 28:1616, 1990.

West, BC and Kwon-Chung, KJ: Mycetoma caused by *Microsporum audouinii.* Am J Clin Pathol 73:447, 1980.

INTRODUCTION

Superficial and cutaneous fungi are often grouped together, since they infect the same outer areas of the body—skin, hair, and nails. **Superficial mycoses** are noninvasive and basically asymptomatic, involving just the top keratin-containing layers of skin or hair, while **cutaneous mycoses** (or **dermatomycoses**) affect the deeper epidermal layers, producing more tissue destruction and symptoms. Primary cutaneous mycoses are caused by *Candida* sp. or the dermatophytes *Microsporum, Epidermophyton,* and *Trichophyton.* The term **tinea,** or ringworm, has been applied traditionally to the diseases elicited by the last three organisms. However, it has been suggested recently that this term be replaced by the term **dermatophytosis,** followed by the body area affected (e.g., tinea capitis should be replaced by **dermatophytosis of the scalp**).

If the skin is abraded, systemic pathogens, for example, *Coccidioides immitis,* also may rarely produce cutaneous infections without involving the rest of the body. In addition, systemic organisms may exhibit secondary cutaneous manifestations as part of the disseminated disease process. Secondary infections must be carefully differentiated from primary ones, as the prognosis and treatment are quite different. Dermatophyte identification is presented in this module; *Candida* and systemic fungus identification is presented in Modules 5 and 7, respectively.

SUPERFICIAL ORGANISMS

Superficial fungi are primarily observed in tropical climates. However, because they are sometimes seen in the United States, they are included in this text. Skin scrapings and plucked hairs are the specimens of choice. See Module 2 for specimen collection and processing. Key identifying features are in capital letters.

**EXOPHIALA
(PHAEOANNEL-
LOMYCES,
CLADOSPORIUM)
WERNECKII**
(Figs. 4–1 and 4–2)

Culture: On SABHI agar at room temperature, a BLACK, YEASTY colony slowly develops, which later may be covered with short olive-gray mycelium (see Color Plate 34).

Microscopic: The yeast portion of the colony contains only DARK, one- or two-celled blastoconidia (Fig. 4–2A). In the older mold portion, hyphae develop with one- or two-celled dark blastoconidia in large clusters (Fig. 4–2B) which resemble *Candida,* and blastoconidia in small clusters (Fig. 4–2C), which resemble the opportunist *Aureobasidium.* Very old colonies produce ANNELLIDES with CLUSTERS or chains of one- or two-celled dark ANNELLOCONIDIA (Fig. 4–2D).

Other comments: It was suggested that *E. wernickii* be reclassified in the genus *Phaeoannelomyces* on the basis of the production of budding cells with annellides when grown on potato dextrose agar at 25°C. However, other morphologic forms may predominate under different culture conditions and media; therefore, the reclassification of this organism into the genus *Phaeoannellomyces* is not accepted by some mycologists (Kwon-Chung and Bennett, 1992).

    E. wernickii may be easily mistaken for *E. jeanselmei* or *Wangiella dermatitidis* (see Module 6). However, these organisms may be differentiated on the basis of nitrate utilization and maximum growth temperature (page 175).

Pathogenicity: Exophiala wernickii causes tinea nigra in which brown to black, nonscaly patches form primarily on the palms of the hands and enlarge over a period of months to years (see Color Plate 35). Most cases in the United States occur in Southeastern states, such as Louisiana, Alabama, and North Carolina. With daily use of topical antifungal agents such as undecylenic acid or an imidazole, the patches usually disappear in 2 to 4 weeks.

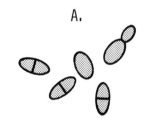

A.

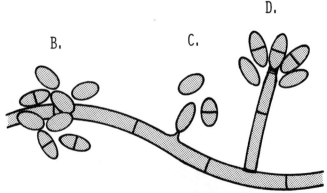

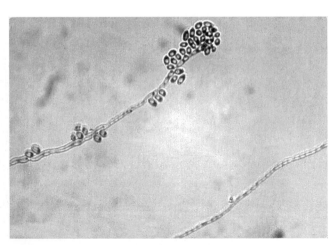

Figure 4–1. *Exophiala werneckii,* lactophenol cotton blue (LPCB) stain (magnification ×450).

Figure 4–2. *Exophiala werneckii.* Figure A: one to two-celled blastoconidia. Figure B: blastoconidia in large clusters resembling *Candida.* Figure C: blastoconidia in small clusters resembling *Aureobasidium.* Figure D: annellides with clusters of annelloconidia.

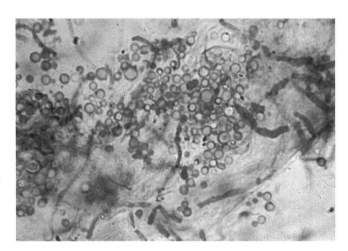

Figure 4–3. *Malassezia furfur,* skin scales, periodic acid–Schiff (PAS) stain. (From Dolan, D, et al: Atlas of Clinical Mycology. ASCP, Washington, DC, 1975, with permission.)

MALASSEZIA FURFUR (PITYROSPORUM OVALE, PITYROSPORUM ORBICULARE) (Figs. 4–3, 4–4, and 4–5)

Culture: M. furfur will not grow on routine culture media unless a lipid such as olive oil is layered over it and the culture is incubated at 37°C. Laboratory diagnosis is confirmed by observing growth of yeast on medium (SABHI or blood agar) overlaid with olive oil or on Faergemann agar (Remel), versus absence of growth on medium without olive oil. The Dupont Isolator system is recommended for recovery of *M. furfur* from blood. Alternatively, addition of 3% palmitic acid to the BACTEC Peds Plus blood culture bottles allows detection of *M. furfur* within 24 to 48 hours with the BACTEC NR 660 system (Nelson et al, 1995).

Microscopic: In KOH or stained preparations from skin disease, *M. furfur* appears as thick, round to oval cells in clusters, accompanied by short, angular hyphae—a SPAGHETTI AND MEATBALLS semblance (Figs. 4–3 and 4–4).

In patients with sepsis, the organism can rarely be seen on smears of peripheral blood. When recovered in laboratory culture, budding yeast cells are observed. Buds form repeatedly from the same pole of the mother cell (UNIPOLAR), resulting in a "collarette" formation (Fig. 4–5).

Pathogenicity: This organism causes **pityriasis versicolor,** an asymptomatic skin infection characterized by scaly patches of different colors: reddish brown, brown, and white (see Color Plate 36). The patches fluoresce under a Wood's lamp. *Malassezia* has also been reported from a case of nasal sinusitis, and from cases of folliculitis (particularly an antibiotic-resistant form occurring on the trunk and legs of AIDS patients) and intravenous line sepsis in patients receiving intravenous lipid infusions (especially premature infants of very low birth weight). Topical application of selenium sulfide or a cream of clotrimazole or miconazole is usually effective therapy for pityriasis versicolor. For treatment of systemic disease, *M. furfur* is susceptible to miconazole and ketaconazole and moderately susceptible to amphotericin B, but resistant to flucytosine.

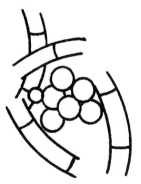

Figure 4–4. *Malassezia furfur.*

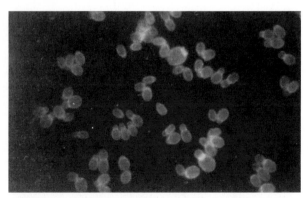

Figure 4–5. *Malassezia furfur* from culture, calcofluor white stain. (From Teglia, O, et al: Infect Control Hosp Epidemiol 12(11):676–681, 1991, with permission.)

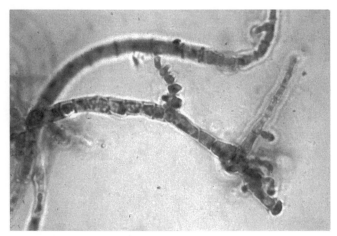

Figure 4–6. *Piedraia hortai.* (From Dolan, D, et al: Atlas of Clinical Mycology. ASCP, Washington, DC, 1975, with permission.)

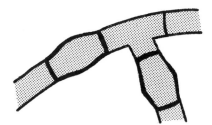

Figure 4–7. *Piedraia hortai.*

PIEDRAIA HORTAI
(Figs. 4–6 through 4–8)

Culture: On SABHI agar at room temperature, a compact, greenish black, heaped, glabrous colony slowly forms.

Microscopic: P. hortai produces DARK, THICK-WALLED HYPHAE with swellings. ASCI containing ascospores may be present.

Pathogenicity: P. hortai causes **black piedra** (Fig. 4–8), which consists of firmly attached, hard black nodules around the outside of scalp hairs. Treatment consists of cutting or shaving all the hairs in the affected area.

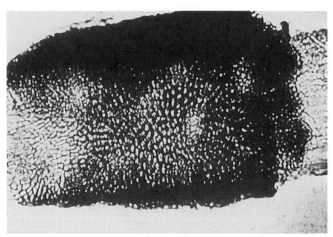

Figure 4–8. Black piedra on hair, high power. (Courtesy of Dr. Leanor Haley, Centers for Disease Control, Atlanta.)

**TRICHOSPORON
BEIGELII
(CUTANEUM)**
(Figs. 4–9 and 4–10)

Culture: On SABHI agar at room temperature, a cream-colored, wrinkled, glabrous colony forms within 5 days (see Color Plate 37).

Microscopic: On corn meal-Tween 80 agar, hyaline hyphae with BLASTOCONIDIA and ARTHROCONIDIA are observed. Biochemical tests can be performed to identify this fungus (see Module 5).

Pathogenicity: Trichosporon beigelii produces **white piedra,** which consists of light brown, soft nodules around beard and mustache hairs (see Color Plate 38). These nodules are less firmly attached than those of black piedra. In immunocompromised patients, invasion of the blood, kidneys, lungs, and skin may occur. This disseminated form of disease usually manifests as fever, pulmonary infiltrates, and cutaneous lesions. Treatment of white piedra consists of cutting or shaving all the hairs in the affected area. In addition, topical application of clotrimazole cream, amphotericin B lotion or 5% ammoniated mercury ointment is recommended to prevent recurrence of the infection. When causing disseminated disease, *T. beigelii* is resistant to amphotericin B (Walsh et al, 1990).

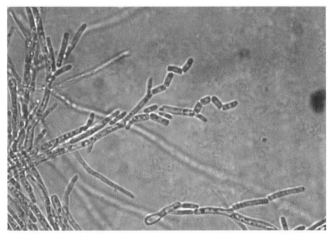

Figure 4–9. *Trichosporon beigelii,* corn meal–Tween 80 (CM-T80) agar (magnification ×450).

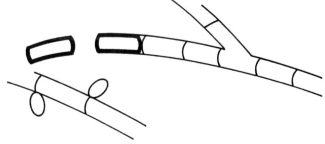

Figure 4–10. *Trichosporon beigelii,* CM-T80.

STUDY QUESTIONS

Matching: Place the letter(s) of the words in Column B in front of the corresponding words in Column A.

Column A

_____ 1. *Trichosporon beigelii*

_____ 2. Spaghetti & meatballs

_____ 3. Black patches on skin

_____ 4. Black piedra

Column B

A. Multicolored patches on skin

B. Tinea nigra

C. Hard, black hair nodules

D. *Malassezia furfur*

E. Light brown hair nodules

F. Black mold mistaken for *Candida* or *Auerobasidium*

STOP HERE UNTIL YOU HAVE COMPLETED THE QUESTIONS.

Look up the answers in the back of the book. If you missed more than one, go back and review the superficial organisms. Correctly complete any missed study questions before proceeding further.

DERMATOPHYTES

Dermatophytes belong to the genera *Microsporum, Epidermophyton,* and *Trichophyton.* **Geophilic** species live in the soil, **zoophilic** species live on animals, and **anthropophilic** species live on humans (Chart 4-1). Not all dermatophytes are pathogenic to humans;

CHART 4–1. ECOLOGICAL CLASSIFICATION OF FREQUENTLY ISOLATED DERMATOPHYTE SPECIES

Anthropophilic	Zoophilic	Geophilic
E. floccosum	M. canis	M. gypseum
M. audouinii	T. mentagrophytes	
T. mentagrophytes	T. verrucosum	
T. rubrum		
T. schoenleinii		
T. tonsurans		
T. violaceum		

Adapted from Tanaka, S, et al: Advances in dermatophytes and dermatophytosis. J Med Vet Mycol 30(Suppl 1):29, 1992.

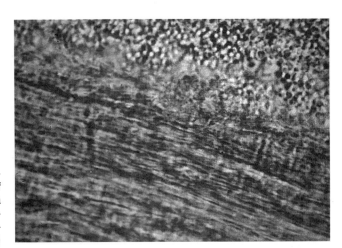

Figure 4–11. Ectothrix hair invasion. Hair shaft is in bottom half of photo and ectothrix arthroconidia are on top. (From Beneke, ES: Human Mycoses, ed. 8, Upjohn, Minneapolis, 1984, with permission.)

one must be aware that nonpathogens may be found as contaminants on specimens. Skin scrapings, nail scrapings, and hair stubs (including the roots) are the usual specimens for dermatophyte study. Potassium hydroxide (KOH) preparations are made and observed for branching septate hyphae in skin and nail scrapings. Addition of calcofluor white to the KOH enhances visualization of hyphal fragments. Staining skin scale specimens with neutral red has been suggested to differentiate viable (positive or red staining) hyphal fragments from nonviable (negative or nonstaining) fragments (Naka et al, 1994). Arthroconidia are sought in hairs, and it is noted whether they are outside the hair shaft (**ectothrix invasion**) or inside (**endothrix invasion**). Be careful in observing hairs, for ectothrix invasion (Fig. 4–11) begins within the shaft at the base and then moves outside further up the hair. Ectothrix and endothrix (Fig. 4–12) characteristics are seen only in direct mounts, not in hairs that have been cultured.

Dermatophyte test medium (DTM) (Oricult, Medical Technology Corp.) is useful as a screening medium. After incubation at room temperature for 14 days, if the organism is a dermatophyte, it will change the yellow indicator to red. There are a few other fungi, for example, *Cladosporium,* that will also change the color of the medium; thus, slide cultures must be performed for definitive identification. SABHI agar with cycloheximide and chloramphenicol is also satisfactory for isolating dermatophytes. (See Module 2 for further details on specimen collection and processing.)

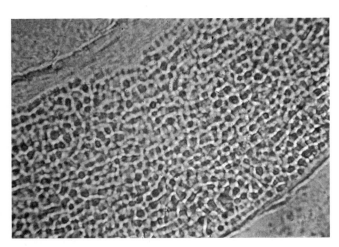

Figure 4–12. Endothrix hair invasion. (From Dolan, D, et al: Atlas of Clinical Mycology. ASCP, Washington, DC, 1975, with permission.)

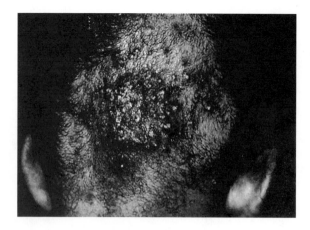

Figure 4–13. Dermatophytosis of the scalp (tinea capitis). (Courtesy of Dr. Robert Kenney, William Beaumont Medical Center, El Paso, TX.)

GENERAL DIFFERENTIAL CHARACTERISTICS

Microsporum, Epidermophyton, and *Trichophyton* may be identified in many different ways.

Location of the Dermatophytosis
(Figs. 4–13 and 4–14)

Dermatophytes infect specific body sites, which are the basis for clinical diagnosis. Location of the dermatophytosis may aid in preliminary fungal identification (Chart 4-2).

Microsporum infects skin and ectothrix hair; *Epidermophyton* invades skin and nails; *Trichophyton mentagrophytes, rubrum,* and *verrucosum* affect skin, nails, and ectothrix hair, while *Trichophyton tonsurans, schoenleinii,* and *violaceum* produce disease in skin, nails, and endothrix hair.

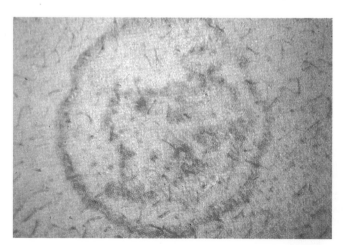

Figure 4–14. Dermatophytosis of the body (tinea corporis). (From Beneke, ES and Rogers, AL: Medical Mycology Manual, ed. 4, Burgess, Minneapolis, 1980, with permission.)

	Skin	Nail	Ectothrix Hair	Endothrix Hair
Microsporum	+		+	
Epidermophyton	+	+		
Trichophyton mentagrophytes rubrum verrucosum	+	+	+	
tonsurans schoenleinii violaceum	+	+		+

Hair Fluorescence Fungi infecting hairs may make a metabolite, pteridine, which produces a bright green-ish yellow fluorescence under a Wood's lamp (366 nm) (see Color Plate 39). Organisms that produce this fluorescence are *Microsporum canis, audouinii, distortum,* and *ferrugineum.* Besides helping to tentatively identify the agent responsible for the infection, fluorescence, if present, will help to choose infected hairs (those that fluoresce) from non-

CHART 4–2. HUMAN DERMATOPHYTOSES AND COMMON CAUSATIVE ORGANISMS*

Dermatophytosis	Other Names	Causative Organisms
Dermatophytosis of the scalp	Tinea capitis	Any *Microsporum* species Any *Trichophyton* (except *T. concentricum*) RARELY *Exophiala werneckii*
Dermatophytosis of the body	Tinea corporis	*M. audouinii, M. canis, M. gypseum* *T. mentagrophytes, T. rubrum, T. verrucosum, T. violaceum* RARELY *T. tonsurans, T. schoenleinii*
Dermatophytosis of the beard	Tinea barbae (barber's itch)	*Microsporum canis* *T. mentagrophytes, T. rubrum, T. verrucosum, T. violaceum*
Dermatophytosis of the groin	Tinea cruris (jock itch)	*Epidermophyton floccosum* *T. mentagrophytes, T. rubrum* *Candida albicans* RARELY *E. werneckii*
Dermatophytosis of the foot	Tinea pedis (athlete's foot)	*E. floccosum* *T. mentagrophytes, T. rubrum* *C. albicans* RARELY *T. tonsurans, T. violaceum, E. werneckii*
Dermatophytosis of the nail	Tinea unguium; onychomycosis	*E. floccosum* *T. mentagrophytes, T. rubrum* *C. albicans* RARELY *T. tonsurans, T. violaceum, T. schoenleinii, M. canis,* *E. werneckii*

* Although *Candida* and *Exophiala* are classified as causing **dermatomycosis** rather than **dermatophytosis,** they may be seen in the same body sites.

infected ones for culture. Note that negative fluorescence of all hairs on the affected body site may still indicate a fungal infection, but by organisms other than those listed above.

Growth Rate

Growth rate is helpful in broadly differentiating the dermatophytes. Of the organisms that commonly elicit symptoms in humans, *Epidermophyton floccosum*, *Microsporum canis*, *Microsporum gypseum*, and *Trichophyton mentagrophytes* form mature colonies in 6 to 10 days (intermediate growers). *Microsporum audouinii*, *Trichophyton rubrum*, *Trichophyton schoenleinii*, *Trichophyton tonsurans*, *Trichophyton verrucosum*, and *Trichophyton violaceum* form mature colonies in 11 to 21 days (slow growers). Another way to remember this is that all the *Microsporum* sp. listed in this module except *M. audouinii* are intermediate growers, while all the *Trichophyton* sp. except *T. mentagrophytes* are slow growers.

Microscopic Characteristics of Each Dermatophyte Genus

For the most important criteria for genus identification refer to Chart 4-3. The microscopic characteristics are rapidly lost with subsequent culture transfers; aerial structures like micro- and macroconidia disappear and only vegetative structures remain. Conidial formation is enhanced by subculturing the organism to media low in nutrients, for example, potato dextrose agar.

With fresh isolates grown on SABHI agar, these are the microscopic characteristics for the dermatophyte genera.

Microsporum sp. produce numerous rough, thick- or thin-walled, elliptical or spindle-shaped macroconidia containing three to seven cells. There are few club-shaped microconidia borne singly along the hyphae. The exception is *M. audouinii*, which rarely produces macro- or microconidia.

Epidermophyton contains only one pathogenic species, *E. floccosum*, which develops numerous smooth, thin-walled, club-shaped macroconidia containing two to four cells. Microconidia are absent.

Trichophyton sp. usually form rare thin-walled, pencil-shaped macroconidia containing three to eight cells; some strains produce numerous macroconidia. Numerous round, oval, or club-shaped microconidia are borne in grapelike clusters or singly along

CHART 4-3. MICROSCOPIC CHARACTERISTICS OF DERMATOPHYTE GENERA

	Microsporum	*Epidermophyton*	*Trichophyton*
Macroconidia:			
Quantity	Numerous	Numerous	Usually rare
Rough- /smooth-walled	Rough	Smooth	Smooth
Shape	Elliptical/spindle	Club	Pencil
Thick- /thin-walled	Thick or thin	Thin	Thin
Number of cells inside	Usually 3–7	Usually 2–4	Usually 3–8
Microconidia:			
Quantity	Few	Absent	Numerous or few
Shape	Club	——	Round, oval, or club
How borne	Singly	——	Singly/grapelike clusters

the hyphae. The exceptions are *T. schoenleinii* and *T. violaceum,* which do not grow macroconidia under ordinary conditions and rarely form microconidia.

Physiologic Tests

Physiologic tests to differentiate the *Microsporum, Trichophyton,* and *Epidermophyton* species have been used, including urease production and assimilation of sugars and nitrogen compounds. Do not confuse these tests with the well-established *Trichophyton* nutritional procedures, which use vitamin requirements for *Trichophyton* sp. differentiation. Of the above tests, urease production is best accepted as a method for differentiating *T. mentagrophytes* from *T. rubrum.*

STUDY QUESTIONS

1. Multiple choice. This is a hair shaft with arthroconidia. The dermatophyte genus which is producing this type of hair invasion is:

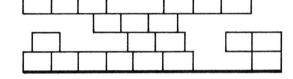

   A. *Microsporum*

   B. *Epidermophyton*

   C. *Candida*

   D. *Trichophyton*

Fill in the blanks:

2. A common name for dermatophytosis of the foot or tinea pedis is _____ .

3. Hair fluorescence is produced from infection with organisms of the _____ genus.

Circle true or false:

4. T F Dermatophytes are usually rapid growers.

5. T F *Epidermophyton* produces no microconidia.

6. Circle the letter(s) of the statement(s) that pertain to the genus *Trichophyton*.

   A. Generally numerous macronidia

   B. Smooth, thin-walled macroconidia

   C. Microconidia in grapelike clusters

   D. Rough, spindle-shaped macroconidia

   E. Numerous or few microconidia

STOP HERE UNTIL YOU HAVE COMPLETED THE QUESTIONS.
If you missed more than one, go back and review the dermatophyte section. Correctly complete any missed study questions before proceeding further.

DERMATOPHYTES PATHOGENIC TO HUMANS

Below are listed specific characteristics of species that cause most of the dermatophytoses in humans. Note that there are many other dermatophytes that rarely infect humans, and also there are many opportunistic dermatophytes that must be differentiated from pathogens. Characteristics especially helpful in identification are in capital letters (Chart 4-4).

Microsporum Species

Microsporum audouinii (Fig. 4–15)

Culture: On SABHI agar at room temperature, a slow-growing, matted to velvety colony forms, which is light tan with a REVERSE color of SALMON (see Color Plates 40 and 41). The salmon color is enhanced if the fungus is cultured on potato dextrose agar. The reverse color tends to turn orange-brown with age; the colony must be observed when it is 1 to 2 weeks old for any salmon color to be present.

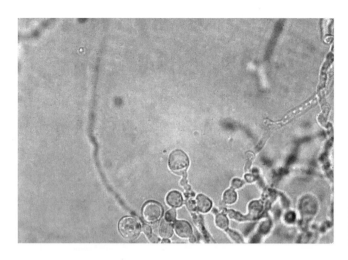

Figure 4–15. Terminal vesicles, *Microsporum audouinii,* LPCB stain (magnification ×450).

CHART 4–4. IDENTIFICATION OF DERMATOPHYTES COMMONLY PATHOGENIC TO HUMANS

I. Macroconidia observed on SABHI agar slide cultures

A. Rough-walled

    1. Thin-walled, numerous   *Microsporum gypseum*

Additional characteristics:
Elliptical, 4- to 6-celled macroconidia
Colony powdery, buff to cinnamon, reverse tan
Few club-shaped microconidia

    2. Thick-walled

      a. Spindle-shaped (tapered ends), numerous   *Microsporum canis*

Additional characteristics:
Macroconidia contain 6 to 15 cells
Colony reverse bright yellow to yellow-orange
Few club-shaped microconidia

      b. Bizarre shaped (aborted), rare   *Microsporum audouinii*

Additional characteristics:
Macroconidia contain 2 to 9 cells
Colony reverse salmon
Prevalent terminal pointed vesicles
Poor growth on rice grains

B. Smooth-walled

    1. Club-shaped, numerous   *Epidermophyton floccosum*

Additional characteristics:
Macroconidia contain 2 to 4 cells
Colony khaki-yellow
No microconidia

    2. Pencil-shaped, rare or numerous

      a.   *Trichophyton mentagrophytes*

Additional characteristics:
Macroconidia contain 5 to 8 cells
Numerous round microconidia, usually in grapelike clusters, although they may appear singly along the hyphae
No red color on potato dextrose agar
Positive urease in 2 to 4 days
Perforates autoclaved hair in vitro

      b.   *Trichophyton rubrum*

Additional characteristics:
Macroconidia contain 3 to 8 cells
Numerous club-shaped microconidia
Red color on potato dextrose agar
Negative urease in 7 days
Does not perforate autoclaved hair in vitro

    3. Aborted, rare   *Trichophyton tonsurans*

Additional characteristics:
Numerous microconidia with great size and shape variation
Grows better in the presence of thiamine

Chart continued on following page

CHART 4–4. IDENTIFICATION OF DERMATOPHYTES COMMONLY
PATHOGENIC TO HUMANS (Continued)

II. Microconidia observed on SABHI agar slide cultures

    A. Numerous microconidia

        1. Grapelike
           clusters,
           round to oval
           cells

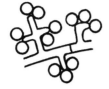

Trichophyton mentagrophytes

Additional characteristics:
Microconidia most commonly in grapelike
    clusters, although they may appear singly
    along the hyphae
Rare or numerous, 5- to 8-celled, pencil-
    shaped, smooth-walled macroconidia
No red color on potato dextrose agar
Positive urease in 2 to 4 days
Perforates autoclaved hair in vitro

        2. Borne singly
           along the hyphae

           a. Uniform size
              and shape

              1.

Trichophyton mentagrophytes

Additional characteristics:
Microconidia most commonly round to oval
    and in grapelike clusters
Rare or numerous, 5- to 8-celled, pencil-
    shaped, smooth-walled macroconidia
No red color on potato dextrose agar
Positive urease in 2 to 4 days
Perforates autoclaved hair in vitro

              2.

Trichophyton rubrum

Additional characteristics:
Rare or numerous, 3- to 8-celled, pencil-
    shaped, smooth-walled macroconidia
Red color on potato dextrose agar
Negative urease in 7 days
Does not perforate autoclaved hair in vitro

           b. Great size and
              shape variation

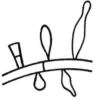

Trichophyton tonsurans

Additional characteristics:
Rare, aborted, smooth-walled macroconidia
Grows better in the presence of thiamine

    B. Few microconidia, club
       shaped

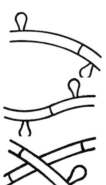

        1. Colony cinnamon,
           reverse tan

Microsporum gypseum

Additional characteristics:
Numerous rough, thin-walled, elliptical
    macroconidia containing 4 to 6 cells

        2. Colony white with
           yellow periphery,
           reverse bright yellow

Microsporum canis

Additional characteristics:
Numerous rough, thick-walled, spindle-shaped
    macroconidia with 6 to 15 cells

    C. Rare microconidia, club
       shaped

Microsporum audouinii

Additional characteristics:
Colony light tan with salmon reverse
Rare, rough, thick-walled, aborted
    macroconidia
Prevalent terminal pointed vesicles
Poor growth on polished rice grains

Chart continued on following page

CHART 4–4. IDENTIFICATION OF DERMATOPHYTES COMMONLY
PATHOGENIC TO HUMANS (Continued)

III. No microconidia or macroconidia observed on SABHI agar slide cultures

			Additional characteristics:
A. Terminal pointed vesicles		*Microsporum audouinii*	Colony light tan with salmon reverse Rare, rough, thick-walled, aborted macroconidia, whose growth is enhanced on media with yeast extract Rare club-shaped microconidia borne singly along the hyphae Common racquet hyphae, nodular bodies Poor growth on polished rice grains
B. Chlamydoconidia in chains			**Additional characteristics:**
1. Colony violet, reverse lavender	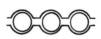	*Trichophyton violaceum*	No macroconidia produced Few microconidia form on thiamine-enriched media Grows better in the presence of thiamine
2. Colony white to bright yellow, reverse nonpigmented to yellow	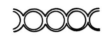	*Trichophyton verrucosum*	**Additional characteristics:** On thiamine-enriched media, rare smooth-walled, rat-tail macroconidia, and moderate club-shaped microconidia are produced Grows better at 37°C Requires thiamine for growth Most strains also require inositol for growth
C. Favic chandeliers prevalent		*Trichophyton schoenleinii*	**Additional characteristics:** Colony light yellow to buff, reverse nonpigmented to yellow-orange No macroconidia produced Chlamydoconidia and hyphal swellings common Microconidia form on rice grains Does not require thiamine for growth

Microscopic: Rare, irregularly shaped macroconidia exhibit thick, rough walls with two to nine cells. Rare club-shaped microconidia are borne singly along the hyphae. Racquet hyphae, nodular bodies, and TERMINAL, usually POINTED, VESICLES (mistaken for chlamydoconidia) are most commonly found.

Other comments: Infected hairs fluoresce. POOR GROWTH on STERILE POLISHED RICE GRAINS (see box) helps differentiate *M. audouinii* from other *Microsporum* species, which grow well on rice grains. Adding yeast extract to the slide culture medium may enhance macroconidial production.

Pathogenicity: M. audouinii causes dermatophytosis of the body and scalp (tinea corporis and children's epidemics of tinea capitis). There has been one reported case of myce-toma produced by this fungus.

RICE GRAINS TEST

Medium Preparation
(Commercially available from Remel)
    Polished unfortified white rice*   8.0 g
    Distilled water   25.0 mL
1. Mix together the rice and water in a small screw-capped bottle.
2. Autoclave at 15 psi for 15 minutes and cool.

Procedure
1. Inoculate the rice surface with two or three fungal fragments, being careful not to carry over any agar from the original tube.
2. Incubate the bottle with the cap loose at room temperature for 8 to 10 days and observe for growth. *M. audouinii* grows poorly on this medium, while other *Microsporum* species proliferate.

*If fortified, make sure the vitamin content of the rice is less than 10% of the Minimum Daily Requirement.

Microsporum canis (Fig. 4–16)

Culture: On SABHI agar at room temperature, a white, woolly colony with a buff to brown center and bright yellow periphery is formed within 1 week. The REVERSE is BRIGHT YELLOW to YELLOW ORANGE (see Color Plates 42 and 43).

Microscopic: There are numerous rough, thick-walled, SPINDLE-SHAPED (tapered ends) MACROCONIDIA containing 6 to 15 cells. A few one-celled, club-shaped microconidia are borne singly along the hyphae. Racquet hyphae, nodular bodies, and chlamydoconidia may be present.

Other comments: Infected hairs fluoresce. Macroconidial production is enhanced by growth on Emmon's medium or modified corn meal agar.

Pathogenicity: M. canis causes dermatophytosis of the body and scalp, which usually are contracted from infected dogs and cats. Invasive infections have been reported in immunosuppressed patients.

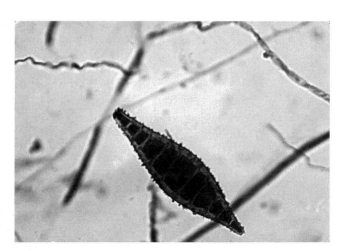

Figure 4–16. Macroconidium, *Microsporum canis,* LPCB stain (magnification ×450).

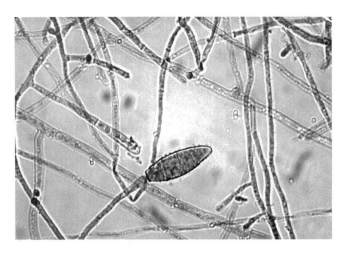

Figure 4–17. Macroconidia and microconidia, *Microsporum gypseum*, LPCB stain (magnification ×450).

Microsporum gypseum (Fig. 4–17)

Culture: On SABHI agar at room temperature, a powdery, BUFF to CINNAMON colony with a tan reverse forms within 1 week (see Color Plate 5).

Microscopic: There are numerous rough, THIN-WALLED, ELLIPTICAL MACROCONIDIA containing four to six cells. A few club-shaped microconidia are borne singly along the hyphae.

Pathogenicity: M. gypseum causes inflammatory dermatophytosis of the body or scalp contracted through contact with contaminated soil.

Epidermophyton Species

Epidermophyton floccosum (Fig. 4–18)

Culture: On SABHI agar at room temperature, a velvety, KHAKI-YELLOW colony with a tan reverse forms within 10 days (see Color Plate 7).

Microscopic: There are numerous CLUB-SHAPED, smooth, thin-walled MACROCONIDIA containing two to four cells. The macroconidia are borne singly or in clusters. No microconidia develop; racquet hyphae, spiral hyphae, nodular bodies, and chlamydoconidia may be present.

Other comments: Macroconidial formation may be enhanced by growing the organism on media with a low sugar content.

Pathogenicity: E. floccosum causes epidemic dermatophytosis (athlete's foot) in summer camps and institutions, as well as dermatophytosis of the nails and groin.

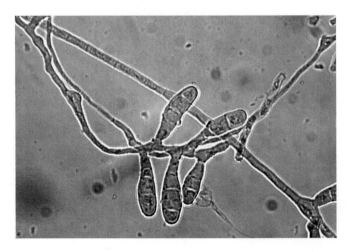

Figure 4–18. Macroconidia, *Epidermophyton floccosum*, LPCB stain (magnification ×450).

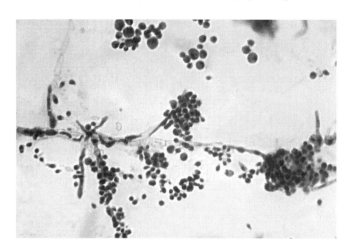

Figure 4–19. Grapelike clusters of microconidia, *Trichophyton mentagrophytes,* LPCB stain (magnification ×450).

Trichophyton Species

The *Trichophyton* species are divided here into groups based on the type of hair invasion. Keep in mind that these fungi also infect skin and nails.

Ectothrix Hair Invasion
Trichophyton mentagrophytes (Figs. 4–19 and 4–20)

Culture: On SABHI agar at room temperature, two colonial textures are seen after 7 to 10 days. Fluffy colonies are white with a colorless to yellow reverse (see Color Plate 44). Granular colonies are buff to rose-tan with a brown, red, or yellow reverse (see Color Plate 45). Red strains may be mistaken for *Trichophyton rubrum.*

Microscopic: Granular forms usually produce numerous pencil-shaped, smooth, thin-walled macroconidia containing five to eight cells, while fluffy strains demonstrate rare macroconidia. Numerous to few ROUND MICROCONIDIA are found in GRAPELIKE CLUSTERS. Microconidia may also be seen singly along the hyphae, but then they are more tear- to club-shaped. Racquet hyphae, spiral hyphae, nodular bodies, and chlamydoconidia may also be present.

Other comments: T. *mentagrophytes* must be differentiated from *T. rubrum;* the former usually forms NO RED PIGMENT on potato dextrose or corn meal agar. It also produces a POSITIVE UREASE reaction in 2 to 4 days on Christenson's urea agar at room temperature, while other dermatophytes may be positive after 5 days. T. *mentagrophytes* PERFORATES AUTOCLAVED HAIR in vitro (see box), although other dermatophytes will too. All three tests must be performed in conjunction with each other for a valid interpretation.

Pathogenicity: T. *mentagrophytes* causes inflammatory dermatophytosis of the foot, body, nails, beard, and scalp. It is the most common cause of athlete's foot.

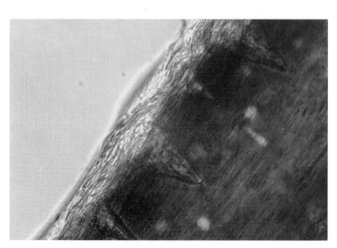

Figure 4–20. Wedge-shaped hair perforations, *Trichophyton mentagrophytes,* LPCB stain (magnification ×450).

IN VITRO HAIR PERFORATION TEST

Medium Preparation

10% yeast extract, filter sterilized	0.1 mL
Sterile distilled water	25.0 mL
Autoclaved healthy human hair, not color-treated or hair sprayed; 1 cm long	Several pieces

1. In a sterile Petri dish, mix the yeast extract and water.
2. Add several pieces of hair.

Procedure

1. Inoculate the hairs in the Petri dish with small bits of fungus to be tested.
2. Cover the dish and incubate at room temperature for 4 weeks.
3. Periodically remove a piece of hair, place with a drop of lactophenol cotton blue on a slide, put on a coverslip, and examine under the microscope for wedge-shaped clear areas (PERFORATIONS) at 90-degree angles to the hair shaft.

    Other organisms besides *T. mentagrophytes* will perforate hair, so do not use this test as the sole basis for differentiating *T. mentagrophytes* from *T. rubrum*.

Trichophyton rubrum (Fig. 4–21)

Culture: On SABHI agar at room temperature, a granular or fluffy white colony with a pink periphery and DEEP RED REVERSE forms in 2 weeks (see Color Plates 46 and 47). The color is best seen on potato dextrose or corn meal agar.

Microscopic: Numerous or few smooth-walled, pencil-shaped macroconidia with three to eight cells are observed. Numerous club-shaped microconidia are borne singly along the hyphae. Chlamydoconidia, racquet hyphae, and nodular bodies may also be present.

Other comments: T. rubrum produces a DEEP RED PIGMENT on potato dextrose or corn meal agar, is UREASE NEGATIVE within 7 days, and DOES NOT PERFORATE AUTO-CLAVED HAIR. Growth on heart infusion tryptose agar greatly enhances macroconidial formation.

Pathogenicity: T. rubrum causes dermatophytosis of the body, foot, groin and nails. In patients receiving immunosuppressive therapy, *T. rubrum* may cause subcutaneous nodules or abscesses.

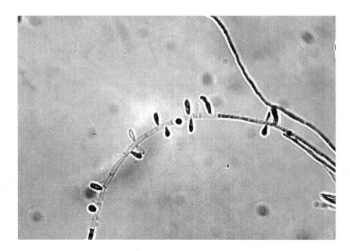

Figure 4–21. Microconidia, *Trichophyton rubrum*, LPCB stain (magnification ×450).

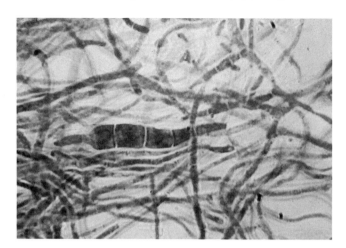

Figure 4–22. Rat-tail macroconidium, *Trichophyton verrucosum.* (From Dolan, D, et al: Atlas of Clinical Mycology. ASCP, Washington, DC, 1975, with permission.)

Trichophyton verrucosum (Fig. 4–22)

Culture: On SABHI agar at room temperature, this organism does not flourish (see Color Plate 48). *T. verrucosum* colonies grow more readily on SABHI agar with yeast extract or on heart infusion tryptose agar with thiamine. On these enriched media at 37°C, a heaped, waxy, white to bright yellow colony with a nonpigmented to yellow reverse forms in 2 to 3 weeks.

Microscopic: On SABHI agar, only chlamydoconidia in chains are produced. On thiamine-enriched media, rare three- to five-celled MACROCONIDIA with an elongated, RAT-TAIL END, and moderate numbers of club-shaped microconidia borne along the hyphae are observed.

Other comments: In *Trichophyton* nutritional tests (see box), *T. verrucosum* REQUIRES THIAMINE for growth and some stains also require INOSITOL (Chart 4-5).

Pathogenicity: *T. verrucosum* causes dermatophytosis of the scalp, beard, or body which usually is acquired from contact with cattle.

TRICHOPHYTON NUTRITIONAL TEST

Media
Commercially available (Difco, Remel)
    Basal Medium + Casein
    Basal Medium + Casein + Thiamine
    Basal Medium + Casein + Inositol
    Basal Medium + Casein + Inositol + Thiamine

Procedure
1. Bring media to room temperature. Pick a tiny, uniform amount of the test fungus from SABHI. Be careful not to take any SABHI along with the fungus, as nutrients may be carried over to the test.
2. Inoculate each *Trichophyton* agar in the center and incubate at 25°C for 2 weeks. If *T. verrucosum* or *T. schoenleinii* is suspected, incubate the agars at 37°C.
3. See Chart 4-5 for the amount of growth on each medium, by species.

CHART 4–5. *TRICHOPHYTON* NUTRITIONAL GROWTH PATTERNS

	Casein Basal Agar	Casein + Inositol	Casein + Inositol + Thiamine	Casein + Thiamine
T. verrucosum (37°C)				
84%	0	±	4+	0
16%	0	0	4+	4+
T. tonsurans	±–1+	2+	4+	4+
T. violaceum	±–1+	1+	4+	4+
Organisms in which nutritional patterns are not helpful:				
T. mentagrophytes	4+	4+	4+	4+
T. rubrum	4+	4+	4+	4+
T. schoenleinii (37°C)	4+	4+	4+	4+

4+ = rich abundant growth
1+ = submerged growth of approximately 10 mm
± = no growth or growth of approximately 2 mm
(Adapted from Koneman, EW, et al: Practical Laboratory Mycology, ed 3. Williams & Wilkins, Baltimore, 1985.)

STUDY QUESTIONS

Fill in the statements below with the letter(s) of the appropriate tests. More than one letter may be used per statement.

A. Urease test

B. Polished rice grains test

C. Red pigment on potato dextrose agar

D. *Trichophyton* nutritional agar tests

E. In vitro hair perforation

1. _____ Test(s) that help differentiate *T. mentagrophytes* from *T. rubrum*

2. _____ Test(s) that help differentiate *M. audouinii* from *M. canis*

3. Circle the letter of the correct answer:

Features that distinguish *M. gypseum* from *M. canis* and *M. audouinii* are all of the following *except:*

A. *M. gypseum* macroconidia are thin walled, while *M. canis* and *M. audouinii* are thick walled.

B. *M. gypseum* colony reverse is tan, while *M. canis* is yellow, and *M. audouinii* is salmon.

C. *M. gypseum* macroconidia are smooth walled, while *M. canis* and *M. audouinii* are rough.

D. *M. gypseum* macroconidia are elliptical, while *M. canis* are spindle shaped and *M. audouinii* are irregularly (aborted) shaped.

4. Circle true or false:

T F *E. floccosum* macroconidia may be confused with those of *T. verrucosum.*

STOP HERE UNTIL YOU HAVE COMPLETED THE QUESTIONS.
If you missed more than two, go back and review the *Microsporum, Epidermophyton,* and ectothrix *Trichophyton* sections. Correctly complete any missed questions before proceeding further.

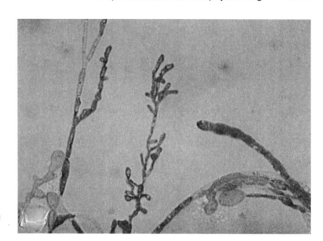

Figure 4–23. Favic chandeliers, *Trichophyton schoenleinii*, LPCB stain (magnification ×450).

Endothrix Hair Invasion

Trichophyton schoenleinii (Fig. 4–23)

Culture: On SABHI agar at room temperature, a waxy, heaped, light yellow to buff colony with a colorless to yellow-orange reverse forms in 2 to 3 weeks (see Color Plate 49).

Microscopic: No macroconidia are exhibited under routine conditions. FAVIC CHANDELIERS are the most prevalent feature; although they may be seen in other species, favic chandeliers are more common in *T. schoenleinii*. Chlamydoconidia and hyphal swellings may be present.

Other comments: Microconidia are formed on rice grains.

Pathogenicity: *T. schoenleinii* causes a severe form of dermatophytosis of the scalp called FAVUS and, rarely, dermatophytosis of the body or nails.

Trichophyton tonsurans (Fig. 4–24)

Culture: On SABHI agar at room temperature, three colonial types are formed in 1 to 2 weeks: a gray-white, suede front with a mahogany reverse; granular white front with a colorless reverse; and a bright yellow, granular to suede, rugose colony with a yellow reverse (see Color Plate 50).

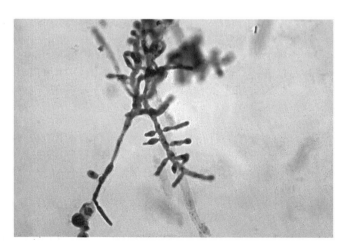

Figure 4–24. Microconidia, *Trichophyton tonsurans*, LPCB stain (magnification ×450).

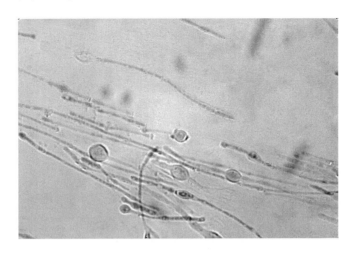

Figure 4–25. Chlamydoconidia, *Trichophyton violaceum*, LPCB stain (magnification ×450).

Microscopic: Rare smooth-walled, club-shaped, or aborted macroconidia are observed. Numerous MICROCONIDIA with a GREAT SIZE and SHAPE VARIATION are seen. Chlamydoconidia and racquet hyphae may be present.

Other comments: Isolates may be confused with *T. mentagrophytes; T. tonsurans* is urease positive after 4 days but does not perforate hair in vitro. In *Trichophyton* nutritional tests, *T. tonsurans* also grows better in the presence of THIAMINE, while *T. mentagrophytes* multiplies well with or without thiamine.

Pathogenicity: T. tonsurans causes over 90% of the cases of dermatophytosis of the scalp (tinea capitis) in the United States today. It is epidemic in black school-age children and may not resolve with puberty. *T. tonsurans* also causes BLACK DOT TINEA CAPITIS (appearance due to broken off hair shafts near the scalp), and occasionally dermatophytosis of the body, foot, and nails.

Trichophyton violaceum (Fig. 4–25)

Culture: On SABHI agar at room temperature, a waxy or suede, VIOLET, heaped colony with a lavender reverse forms in 2 to 3 weeks (see Color Plate 51). The violet color may be lost on subculture. Better growth occurs on SABHI agar with trypticase and thiamine.

Microscopic: Macroconidia are not produced; only chlamydoconidia in chains and hyphal swellings are observed.

Other comments: In *Trichophyton* nutritional tests, *T. violaceum* requires THIAMINE. On thiamine-enriched media, a few microconidia may be formed.

Pathogenicity: T. violaceum causes dermatophytosis of the scalp and body and, rarely, the foot, nails, or deep infections.

DERMATOPHY-TOSIS (TINEA, RINGWORM)

Natural and experimental infection with species of dermatophytes has shown that the course of the infection demonstrates the following sequence (Knudsen, EA, 1989):

1. Week 1: The original follicular lesion is replaced by a circular area of erythema with occasional itching. Positive cultures can be obtained from the central erythema as well as 39 to 40 mm into the normal appearing periphery. By the seventh day of infection, a positive skin test can be detected.
2. Week 2: Satellite lesions may occur, the original lesion peaks in intensity, and positive cultures are obtained as far as 45 mm beyond the edge of the lesion.
3. Week 3: The original lesion reaches its maximum size and begins to heal in the center. Scrapings for culture should be taken only from the outer red ring, not from the healed center. Positive cultures can still be obtained from normal-appearing skin as far as 35 mm outside the visible lesion.
4. Weeks 4 and 5: Central healing continues and cultures from the normal-appearing peripheral skin are negative.

5. Week 6: Cultures from the central lesion and surrounding skin are negative. The affected skin slowly returns to normal as the lesion heals.

In the immunocompetent host, dermatophytosis is limited to the keratinized, horny layers of the skin, hair, and nails and follows the sequence described above. However, in patients with impaired immune function due to disease (e.g., AIDS) or immunosuppressive therapy, the infection may become chronic, or lesions may extend into the subcutaneous, or more rarely, deep-seated tissues.

When zoophilic species of dermatophytes are isolated, pets of the patient should be examined because they may serve as a vector for the infection. Although infection may not be apparent, the pet should be treated as well as the patient. When anthropophilic species are isolated, other family members or close personal contacts should be examined and treated if infected.

Appropriate therapy for dermatophytosis is dependent on the location on the infection. Mild cases of dermatophytosis of the foot, body, and groin are treated effectively with topical agents such as the azoles. However, dermatophytes of the scalp, extensive cases of dermatophytosis of the body, and subcutaneous infections should be treated systemically with griseofulvin. Dermatophytosis of the nails requires prolonged therapy (3 to 12 months) with griseofulvin or itraconazole.

FINAL EXAM

1. Superficial and cutaneous mycoses are similar in that they involve skin and hair. How do they differ?

2. Circle true or false:

   T   F   All dermatophytes infecting humans cause cutaneous mycoses, but not all cutaneous mycoses are elicited by dermatophytes.

3. Circle the letter of the correct answer:

   This organism is an etiologic agent of epidemic dermatophytosis of the foot in summer camps and institutions. It does not infect hair.

   A. *Trichophyton mentagrophytes*

   B. *Epidermophyton floccosum*

   C. *Microsporum audouinii*

   D. *Trichophyton violaceum*

   E. *Trichosporon beigelii*

4. These are the characteristics of a fungus isolated from a patient with dermatophytosis of the scalp:

Culture: (SABHI)	Waxy, buff colony, reverse colorless
Growth rate:	Slow
Slide culture: (SABHI)	Many favic chandeliers, few chlamydoconidia and hyphal swellings

   Circle the letter of the correct answer.

   This organism most likely is:

   A. *Microsporon gypseum*

   B. *Trichophyton tonsurans*

   C. *Trichophyton mentagrophytes*

   D. *Epidermophyton floccosum*

   E. *Tricophyton schoenleinii*

5. *Trichophyton verrucosum* and *Trichophyton violaceum* both may cause dermatophytosis of the scalp, are slow growers, may produce only chlamydoconidia in chains on SABHI agar slide cultures, and are enhanced if grown on media containing yeast extract (has thiamine). How may these fungi be differentiated? Give at least two ways.

6. A patient with black nodules on the scalp hairs came to the dermatology clinic. On SABHI agar, a greenish-black, glabrous colony slowly formed. Slide cultures on SABHI agar showed thick, dark-walled, septate hyphae with numerous intercalary swellings. This organism is most likely (circle the letter of the correct answer):

   A. *Trichophyton violaceum*

   B. *Piedraia hortai*

   C. *Trichophyton verrucosum*

   D. *Microsporum audouinii*

   E. *Exophiala werneckii*

Matching: Place the letter of the answer in Column B in front of the words in Column A. Answers may be used more than once.

Column A

7. _____ Dermatophytosis of the nails

8. _____ Variously sized and shaped microconidia

9. _____ Microconidia in grapelike clusters

10. _____ Salmon colony reverse

11. _____ Hairs fluoresce

12. _____ (+) Urease in 2 to 4 days

Column B

A. *Dermatophytosis of the foot*

B. *Microsporum audouinii*

C. *Trichophyton tonsurans*

D. *Trichophyton mentagrophytes*

E. Tinea unguium

F. *Trichophyton rubrum*

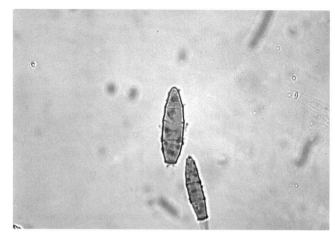

Figure 4–26. Final examination demonstration, LPCB stain (magnification ×450).

13. See Figure 4–26. These macroconidia are characteristic of:

    A. *Microsporum canis*

    B. *Microsporum audouinii*

    C. *Epidermophyton floccosum*

    D. *Trichophyton rubrum*

    E. *Microsporum gypseum*

STOP HERE UNTIL YOU HAVE COMPLETED THE QUESTIONS.

If you missed more than three, go back and repeat this module. Correctly complete any missed questions.

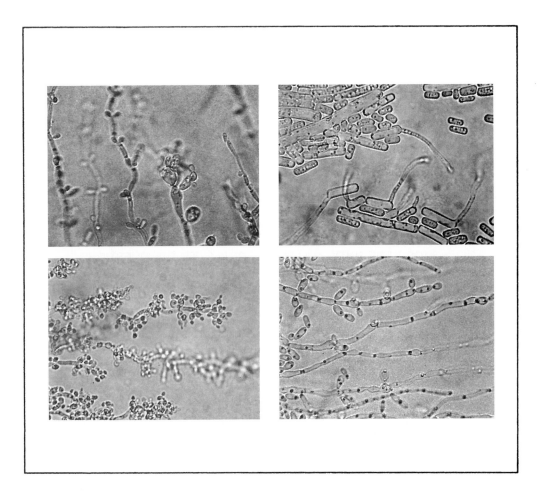

MODULE

5

Yeasts

PREREQUISITES

The learner must possess a good background knowledge in clinical microbiology and must have finished Module 1, Basics of Mycology, and Module 2, Laboratory Procedures for Fungal Culture and Isolation.

BEHAVIORAL OBJECTIVES

Upon completion of this module, the learner should be able to:

1   Identify, from colonial morphology, corn meal-Tween 80 morphology, and appropriate biochemical tests:

Candida albicans
Candida tropicalis
Candida parapsilosis
Candida pseudotropicalis
Candida krusei
Candida guilliermondii
Other *Candida* species
Trichosporon species, including *T. beigelii*

Geotrichum species, including
    G. candidum
Rhodotorula species
Cryptococcus species, including
    C. neoformans
Saccharomyces species
Torulopsis glabrata

2   Correctly perform and interpret results from the following, including when to use each:

Corn meal-Tween 80 morphology
Germ tube test
Carbohydrate assimilations
Carbohydrate fermentations
Urease test
Rapid nitrate test
Malt extract for *Trichosporon* and
    Geotrichum blastoconidia

Malt extract agar for ascospores
Modified Kinyoun acid-fast stain
India ink preparation
Caffeic acid or niger seed agar for
    Cryptococcus neoformans

3   Write a schema for identification of each of the organisms in objective number 1.

4   Briefly discuss candidiasis, cryptococcosis, and diseases caused by *Torulopsis glabrata* and *Geotrichum candidum* including etiologic agents, manifestations, disease incidence (common or rare), and mode of transmission.

CONTENT OUTLINE

I. Introduction
II. Laboratory procedures
  A. Direct examination and cultural isolation
  B. Yeast identification methods

1. Germ tube production
2. Microscopic morphology on corn meal-Tween 80 agar
3. Birdseed agar

4. Study questions
5. Biochemical identification
6. Other tests
7. Study questions
III. Yeast diseases
    A. Candidiasis

B. Cryptococcosis
C. Diseases caused by *Geotrichum candidum*
D. Diseases caused by *Torulopsosis glabrata*
IV. Final exam

FOLLOW-UP ACTIVITIES

1 Students may compare colonial morphology of yeasts on *Candida* BCG agar.

2 Students may look under the microscope at corn meal-Tween 80 preparations of various yeasts.

3 Students may be assigned unknown yeasts for which they must perform differential identification tests.

REFERENCES

Bougnoux, ME, et al: Resolutive *Candida utilis* fungemia in a nonneutropenic patient. J Clin Microbiol 31:1644, 1993.

Branchini, ML, et al: Genotypic variation and slime production among blood and catheter isolates of *Candida parapsilosis.* J Clin Microbiol 32:452, 1994.

Crist, AE, et al: Comparison of the MUREX *C. albicans,* Albicans-Sure, and BactiCard *Candida* with the germ tube test for the presumptive identification of *Candida albicans* (abstr). Presented at the annual meeting of the American Society for Microbiology, Washington, DC, May, 1995.

Dealler, S: *Candida albicans* colony identification in 5 minutes in a general microbiology laboratory. J Clin Microbiol 29:1081, 1991.

Dooley, DP, et al: Misidentification of clinical yeast isolates by using the updated Vitek yeast biochemical card. J Clin Microbiol 32:2889, 1994.

El-Zaatari, M, et al: Evaluation of the updated Vitek yeast identification data base. J Clin Microbiol 28:1938, 1990.

Fenn, JP, et al: Comparison of updated Vitek yeast biochemical card and API 20C yeast identification systems. J Clin Microbiol 32:1184, 1994.

Gurevitz, O, et al: *Cryptococcus neoformans* vertebral osteomyelitis. J Med Vet Mycol 32:315, 1994.

Hadfield, TL, et al: Mycoses caused by *Candida lusitaniae.* Rev Infect Dis 9:1006, 1987.

Land, G, et al: Evaluation of the Baxter Micro-Scan four-hour based yeast identification system. J Clin Microbiol 29:718, 1991.

Marler, JK and Enriquez, LA: Comparison of the IDS RapID Yeast Plus System and the API 20C for the identification of medically important yeast (abstr). Presented at the annual meeting of the American Society for Microbiology, Washington, DC, May, 1995.

Molina, SC, et al: A microfermentation test for the rapid identification of yeasts. J Med Vet Mycol 30:323, 1992.

Nielson, H, et al: *Candida norvegensis* peritonitis and invasive disease in a patient on continuous ambulatory peritoneal dialysis. J Clin Microbiol 28:1664, 1990.

Odds, FC and Bernaerts, R: CHROMagar *Candida,* a new differential isolation medium for presumptive identification of clinically important *Candida* species. J Clin Microbiol 32:1923, 1994.

Perry, J, et al: Rapid colorimetric identification of *Candida albicans.* J Clin Microbiol 28:614, 1990.

Pfaller, A, et al: *Candida zeylanoides:* another opportunistic yeast. J Clin Microbiol 29:1689, 1991.

Shankland, G, et al: Multicenter evaluation of Microring YT, a new method of yeast identification. J Clin Microbiol 28:2808, 1990.

St Germain, G and Beauchesne, D: Evaluation of the Micro-Scan rapid yeast ID panel. J Clin Microbiol 29:2296, 1991.

Warnock, DW and Richardson, MD: Fungal infection in the compromised patient, ed 2. John Wiley & Sons, New York, 1991.

INTRODUCTION   *Candida albicans* and *Cryptococcus neoformans* are the most important yeasts associated with human disease. New technologies have emerged allowing cryptococcal and candidal antigen detection directly from clinical specimens (see Seromycology, Module 2). Although these remain the most common yeast pathogens, unusual strains are being seen more frequently as infectious agents, especially in AIDS patients, transplant and cancer patients, and patients on corticosteroids. Because of the rapid onset of illness in these people, emphasis has been placed on rapid identification of the causative agent. Yeast speciation relies heavily on biochemical identification; thus it lends itself nicely to commercial kits and automated rapid identification systems. These will be discussed in this module.

LABORATORY PROCEDURES

DIRECT EXAMINATION AND CULTURAL ISOLATION

Yeasts may be isolated from almost any specimen. Saline wet preparations of the specimen will show round to oval budding cells (blastoconidia), and some cells may be elongated, forming pseudohyphae. Occasionally, arthroconidia, asci, or other structures are observed.

Capsules may be seen around yeast cells on India ink preparations, suggesting *C. neoformans*. However, other yeasts (*Rhodotorula*, other *Cryptococcus* sp.) may produce capsules, whereas *C. neoformans* may lack them. (See Module 2 for specimen collection and direct examination procedures.)

Yeasts are best grown at 25 to 30°C on SABHI agar. Incorporation of cycloheximide in the medium, or a 37°C incubation inhibits many strains. In 2 or 3 days, yeasts form cream-colored (rarely, orange), glabrous colonies that are mucoid or waxy and smooth or wrinkled.

Most yeasts grow on standard bacteriology sheep blood agar plates and, when young, yeast colonies may be mistaken for *Staphylococcus* sp. Additionally, yeasts are catalase-positive and coagulase-negative like *S. epidermidis*. Yeasts may also grow on bacteriology EMG agar, macroscopically resembling gram-negative rod-shaped bacteria. Always verify the colony by Gram stain or LPCB mount.

YEAST IDENTIFICATION METHODS

Once the yeast is isolated on primary nonselective media, a germ tube test is performed.

Germ Tube Production

In this procedure (see box) one must be careful not to confuse germ tubes with pseudohyphae:

Germ tubes	*Pseudohyphae*
Parallel sides	Not necessarily parallel
Nonseptate	May be septate
No constriction at point of attachment	Constricted

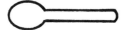 

Germ tubes are formed within 3 hours by *C. albicans* (Fig. 5–1), *C. stellatoidea*, a subspecies of *C. albicans*, and rarely *C. tropicalis*. Other *Candida* strains may produce them

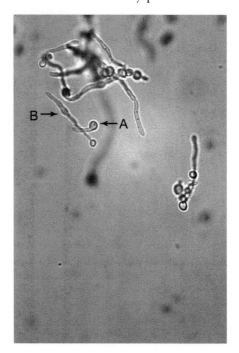

Figure 5–1. *Candida albicans* in human serum after 3 hours' incubation at 37°C (magnification ×450). Arrow A indicates a germ tube; arrow B points to a pseudohypha.

GERM TUBE PRODUCTION

Medium Preparation
1. Place 0.5 mL of rabbit, fetal calf, or human serum into tubes. Rabbit coagulase plasma works well too.

Procedure
1. Inoculate the tube of serum with a small amount of the young test organism. A too-large inoculum will inhibit germ tube formation. Be sure to set up positive and negative controls, particularly if human serum is to be used, to ensure that the serum does not possess anti-*Candida* antibodies and other inhibitory factors.
2. Incubate the tube at 37°C for 3 hours.
3. Place one drop of the suspension on a slide, put on a coverslip, and examine it microscopically for long tubelike projections (germ tubes) extending out from the yeast cells.

---

after 3 hours. Germ tubes may also be produced by arthroconidia, but the arthroconidia should be easily differentiated from blastoconidia. Note that not all *C. albicans* isolates form germ tubes, especially those from cancer patients on therapy or persons on anti-*Candida* antifungals.

If the germ tube test is positive (+), many laboratories stop here and call the organism *C. albicans*. If the germ tube test is negative (−), subculture to (1) corn meal-Tween 80 agar for chlamydospore and specific blastoconidial pattern, (2) birdseed (niger seed, caffeic acid) agar for pigment production of *C. neoformans,* and (3) neutral Sabouraud's agar (Emmon's modification) for later biochemical testing.

Microscopic Morphology on Corn Meal-Tween 80 Agar

Corn meal agar without dextrose should be used, with 0.3% Tween 80 added. It is highly recommended that a separate rice extract agar with 0.3% Tween 80 be used in conjunction with corn meal-Tween 80. Better chlamydospore development occurs on the rice extract medium, while blastoconidial development is enhanced on the corn meal. Tubed media are preferred: they can be freshly melted down as needed and poured into biplates (see box).

MORPHOLOGY ON CORN MEAL-TWEEN 80 AGAR
AND RICE EXTRACT-TWEEN 80 AGAR

Media Preparation
Corn meal-Tween 80 agar (commercially available, Difco, BBL)

Corn meal	50 g
Agar	15 g
Distilled water	1 L
Tween 80	3 mL

Rice extract-Tween 80 agar (commercially available, Difco, BBL)

Cream of rice	10 g
Distilled water	1 L
Agar	10 g
Tween 80	3 mL

1. For the commercial media, follow the manufacturer's instructions regarding reconstitution. Go to number 4.
2. For homemade corn meal-Tween 80 agar, mix the corn meal in 500 mL distilled water, then autoclave at 15 psi for 10 minutes. Filter through cheesecloth, bring the volume to 1 liter with distilled water, and add the agar. Go to number 4.

MORPHOLOGY ON CORN MEAL-TWEEN 80 AGAR AND RICE EXTRACT-TWEEN 80 AGAR (Continued)

3. For homemade rice extract-Tween 80 agar, boil 500 mL of distilled water, add the cream of rice, and cook for 30 seconds. Filter through cheesecloth, bring the volume up to 1 liter with distilled water, and add the agar.
4. Bring the medium to a boil on a hotplate, using a magnetic stirring rod. Add the Tween 80, mixing well.
5. Dispense 10 mL aliquots into screw-capped tubes, autoclave at 15 psi for 15 minutes, cool, and refrigerate.
6. When needed, boil one tube each of corn meal-Tween 80 agar and rice extract-Tween 80 agar, pour into a sterile labeled biplate, and cool.

Procedure
1. Use a very small amount of a young colony. Make two parallel streaks on the agar with an inoculated loop.
2. Flame the loop, then move back and forth across the streaks: DO NOT cut into the agar.
3. Flame a glass coverslip and place it over the inoculated agar. Tamp down on the coverslip with forceps to remove trapped air.
4. After 48 hours at room temperature, remove the Petri dish lid and examine under the coverglass, near the edges, for characteristic features, using the low- and high-power objectives of the microscope. If necessary, reincubate for more growth and examine daily. See Chart 5-1.

If there are chlamydospores, blastoconidia, and pseudohyphae on corn meal-Tween 80 or rice extract-Tween 80 agar, *C. albicans* (Fig. 5–2 and Chart 5-1) is probably the organism in question. It is by far the most commonly isolated yeast in clinical specimens.

C. tropicalis may also rarely produce chlamydospores.* Perform the carbohydrate assimilations for final identification.† Sucrose fermentation may be necessary to rule out *C. tropicalis*.

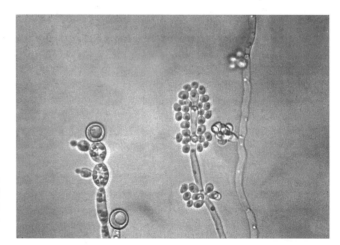

Figure 5–2. Clusters of blastoconidia along the pseudohyphae and terminal chlamydospores, *Candida albicans,* corn meal-Tween 80 (CM-T80) agar (magnification ×450).

---

*If corn meal-Tween 80 plates are incubated at room temperature and then refrigerated for 3 days before reading (for example, over a holiday weekend), *C. tropicalis* will have consistently formed chlamydospores.
†Most, but not all, *C. albicans* form germ tubes and chlamydospores.

CHART 5–1. YEAST MICROSCOPIC MORPHOLOGY ON CORN MEAL–TWEEN 80 AGAR

I. Chlamydospores, blastoconidia, and pseudohyphae

A. Terminal, circular, thick-walled chlamydospores; clusters of numerous or few blastoconidia at septa of pseudohyphae; true hyphae may be present

Candida albicans
Perform germ tube and biochemicals

B. Rare terminal, round or variously shaped, thin-walled chlamydospores; sparse single or short-chained blastoconidia anywhere along the pseudohyphae

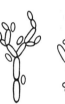

Candida tropicalis
Perform germ tube and biochemicals

II. Blastoconidia and pseudohyphae

A. Oval blastoconidia in chains from the septa of thin pseudohyphae; or clusters of numerous blastoconidia at the septa of short pseudohyphae; often few pseudohyphae produced; great morphologic variation

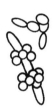

Candida guilliermondi
Perform biochemicals

B. Treelike branching of abundant blastoconidia from the septa of elongated pseudohyphae; alternatively said to have a cross-matchsticks appearance.

Candida krusei
Perform biochemicals

C. Few single or small clustered blastoconidia at or between septa of thin curved pseudohyphae. Sometimes giant pseudohyphae may be observed.

Candida parapsilosis
Perform biochemicals

D. Branched pseudohyphae with chains of elongated blastoconidia at the septa; logs in a stream arrangement of broken up blastoconidia positioned parallel to each other

Candida pseudotropicalis
Perform biochemicals

E. Sparse single or short-chained blastoconidia, at or between septa of pseudohyphae

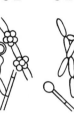
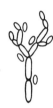

Candida tropicalis
Perform biochemicals

III. Arthroconidia and true hyphae

A. Blastoconidia produced, but they may be difficult to find on corn meal-Tween 80 agar

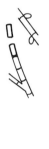

Trichosporon species or *Blastoschizomyces*
Inoculate malt extract broth (observe colonial and microscopic morphology), and perform biochemicals

B. Blastoconidia not produced

← Germ tube

Geotrichum species
Inoculate malt extract broth (observe colonial and microscopic morphology), and perform biochemicals

IV. Blastoconidia only, or with rare short pseudohyphae

A. Pigmented colony on Emmon's agar

1. Pink-orange colony on SABHI agar; corn meal-Tween 80 morphology exhibits oval budding cells with occasional rudimentary pseudohyphae; sometimes a faint capsule is observed

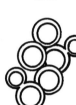

Rhodotorula species or *Sporobolomyces*
Perform biochemicals
Backup: look for satellite colonies produced by *Sporobolomyces* ballistoconidia

B. No colony pigment on Emmon's agar

1. Capsule on India ink preparation

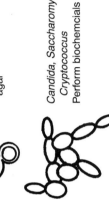

Cryptococcus species
Perform biochemicals and inoculate niger seed or caffeic acid agar

2. No capsule on India ink preparation

Candida, Saccharomyces, Torulopsis, Rhodotorula, Cryptococcus
Perform biochemicals

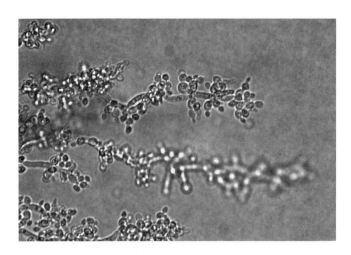

Figure 5–3. Clusters of blastoconidia between short pseudohyphae, *Candida guilliermondi*, CM-T80 agar (magnification ×450).

If blastoconidia and pseudohyphae are produced on corn meal-Tween 80 or rice extract-Tween 80 agar, various *Candida* species may be suspected (Figs. 5–3 through 5–7). The distinctive morphology of each greatly aids in speciation, but perform assimilations for confirmatory identification. If there is still difficulty discerning the species, fermentations may be helpful.

If there are arthroconidia and true hyphae on corn meal-Tween 80 or rice extract-Tween 80 agar, *Trichosporon*, *Blastoschizomyces*, or *Geotrichum* species may be suspected. Occasionally *Trichosporon* or *Blastoschizomyces* may produce blastoconidia, although they may be difficult to find, but *Geotrichum candidum* (Fig. 5–8) does not form blastoconidia. Be careful not to misidentify the corner buds, or germ tubes, extending from some arthroconidia as blastoconidia. To enhance blastoconidial formation, inoculate malt extract broth (same as Wickerham's malt extract agar, page 155, but eliminate agar) with the organism and incubate it at room temperature for 3 to 4 days. Examine a wet mount microscopically for the characteristic budding cells. Perform carbohydrate assimilations for confirmation of the species.

If there are blastoconidia only (or also rare short pseudohyphae) on corn meal-Tween 80 agar or rice extract-Tween 80 agar, *Cryptococcus* (Fig. 5–9), *Rhodotorula*, *Saccharomyces* (Fig. 5–10) or *Candida* species may be suspected. *Rhodotorula* generally produces pink-orange colonies, although it may lose pigment. The uncommon yeast *Sporobolomyces* sp. also possesses a pink-orange color, but on corn meal-Tween 80 agar, blastoconidia, **ballistoconidia** (forcibly ejected conidia on denticles (Fig. 5–11), pseudohyphae, and true hyphae are formed. Additionally, satellite colonies are produced by the ejected ballistoconidia. Both *Rhodotorula* and *Sporobolomyces* resemble the colonies of the *Serratia*

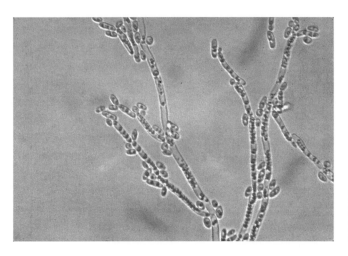

Figure 5–4. "Cross-matchsticks" blastoconidia along pseudohyphae, *Candida krusei*, CM-T80 agar (magnification ×450).

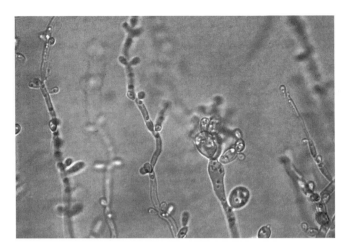

Figure 5–5. Giant and thin curved pseudohyphae, *Candida parapsilosis,* CM-T80 agar (magnification ×450).

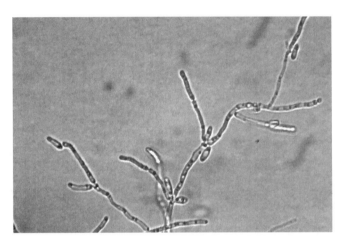

Figure 5–6. "Logs-in-a-stream" blastoconidia along pseudohyphae, *Candida pseudotropicalis,* CM-T80 agar (magnification ×450).

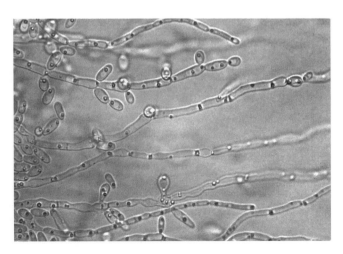

Figure 5–7. Sparse blastoconidia along pseudohyphae, *Candida tropicalis,* CM-T80 agar (magnification ×450).

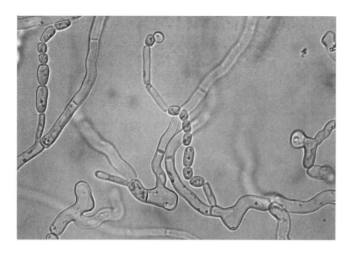

Figure 5–8. Arthroconidia, *Geotrichum candidum,* CM-T80 agar (magnification ×450).

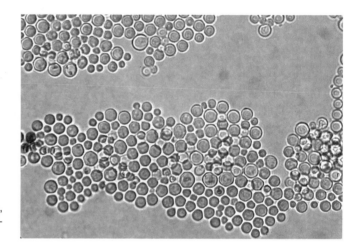

Figure 5–9. Round blastoconidia, *Cryptococcus neoformans,* CM-T80 agar (magnification ×450).

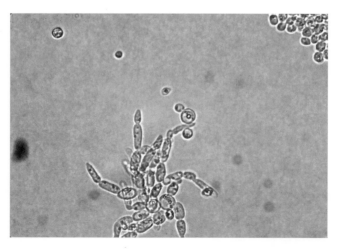

Figure 5–10. Blastoconidia and short pseudohyphae, *Saccharomyces cerevisiae,* CM-T80 agar (magnification ×450).

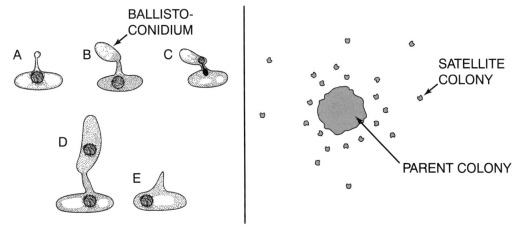

Figure 5–11. *Left:* Development of microscopic ballistoconidia; *Right:* satellite colonies on agar.

bacteria: a Gram stain must be performed to differentiate them. For the nonpigmented yeasts, birdseed agar (for *C. neoformans*) and biochemical panels must be performed for proper identification.

Birdseed Agar

Birdseed (niger seed or caffeic acid) agar is commercially available. After 2 to 3 days of incubation, *C. neoformans* produces dark brown colonies on this medium, whereas other *Cryptococcus* sp. and other yeasts do not (see Color Plate 53).

BIRDSEED (NIGER SEED, *GUIZOTIA ABYSSINICA*) AGAR

Medium Preparation:

Niger seed extract	200 mL
Glucose	1 g
Diphenyl solution (0.1 g/1 mL 95% ethyl alcohol)	10 mL
Agar	20 g
Distilled water	800 mL

Procedure:
1. Niger seed (Philadelphia Seed Co, Philadelphia, PA) is thoroughly pulverized in a blender.
2. 70 g seed powder is added to 350 mL distilled water and autoclaved for 10 min at 121°C.
3. The seed-water extract is filtered through gauze.
4. Combine ingredients under Medium Preparation above.
5. Autoclave for 20 min at 121°C and pour plates.

STUDY QUESTIONS

1. On a vaginal culture, a cream-colored yeast grows on SABHI medium. On corn meal-Tween 80 agar, only small oval blastoconidia are observed. This organism is most likely:

    A. *Candida albicans*

    B. *Trichosporon beigelii*

    C. *Torulopsis glabrata*

    D. *Rhodotorula rubra*

    E. *Geotrichum candidum*

Matching. Place the letter of the answer in **Column B** *in front of the corresponding words in* **Column A.**

Column A	Column B
____ 2. Produces asci	A. *Candida parapsilosis*
____ 3. Logs in a stream blastoconidia	B. *Candida krusei*
____ 4. Thick capsule	C. *Candida pseudotropicalis*
____ 5. Cross-matchsticks blastoconidia	D. *Saccharomyces cerevisiae*
____ 6. Giant pseudohyphae	E. *Geotrichum candidum*
	F. *Cryptococcus neoformans*
	G. *Candida guilliermondii*

7. On corn meal-Tween 80 agar, a fungus produces terminal round chlamydospores and clusters of numerous blastoconidia. The organism also forms germ tubes within 3 hours and assimilates sucrose but does not ferment it. This organism is named _____.

STOP HERE UNTIL YOU HAVE COMPLETED THE QUESTIONS.

Look up the answers in the back of the book. If you missed more than one, go back and review this section. Correctly complete any missed study questions before proceeding further.

BIOCHEMICAL IDENTIFICATION

Today commercial identification panels have taken over the tedious chore of individual assimilations, urease, nitrate, and so forth. Fermentations are reserved as backup only when the commercial systems are not adequate for organism identification. For a discussion of the noncommercial individual biochemical methods, refer to the first edition of this text. Because each commercial panel is constantly changing regarding the biochemicals and data bases included in the kit, a detailed discussion of each kit is not warranted. Refer to the kit package inserts for up-to-date information.

Some manual panels include API 20C and API Rapid Yeast Ident (BioMerieux Vitek), Uni-Yeast-Tek (Flow Labs), Microring YT (Medical Wire and Equipment), RapID Yeast Plus System (distributed by Remel and made by Innovative Diagnostic Systems), and Minitek (BBL).

Automated systems include AutoMicrobic (BioMerieux-Vitek) and MicroScan Rapid Yeast Ident (Baxter). The Quantum (Abbott Laboratories) is phasing out yeast identification.

Some of the manual and automated panels rely on growth and assimilation, with a 2- to 3-day turnaround time. While these tests are more established, newer panels, which detect an enzymatic reaction, give a 4-hour turnaround time (MicroScan Rapid Yeast Ident, Innovative Diagnostics RapID Yeast Plus System, API Yeast Ident). These rapid tests give satisfactory results and may well take over the market in the future.

In addition to panels for detecting yeasts in general, there are commercial kits for identifying *C. albicans* alone. These include the *C. albicans* Screen (Carr-Scarborough), Albistrip (Lab M, Ltd), Smith-Kline Isocult, Bacti-Card *Candida* (Remel), the MUREX *C. albicans* enzyme kit (Murex Diagnostics), and Albicans-Sure (Clinical Standards Laboratories).

There are many articles comparing the accuracy, sensitivity, and specificity of the various commercial kits. These are summarized in Chart 5-2. A list of biochemical reactions for each yeast is in Chart 5-3.

Other Tests

Yeast colonial morphology may sometimes aid in identification. While the birdseed agar for *C. neoformans* is in widespread use, there are other media such as *Candida* BCG (see Color Plate 55), BiGGY, and now CHROMagar (Odds and Bernaerts 1994), which show different colonial characteristics for each yeast.

Additionally, *Saccharomyces* and some other yeasts produce asci, the sexual stage, when grown on Wickerham's malt extract agar. After growth, the organism is smeared on a slide and stained with the modified Kinyoun acid-fast stain (see Module 2). Asci stain red while other yeast cells stain blue (see Color Plate 52).

CHART 5–2. COMPARISON OF COMMERCIAL YEAST IDENTIFICATION KITS

	Test*	Accuracy	Sensitivity	Specificity	Test Comparison	References
C. ALBICANS ONLY	C. albicans screen (Carr-Scarborough)	98.3%			API 20 C	(Perry et al. 1990)
	Albistrip (Lab M Ltd)		98.0%	98.0%	API 20 C	(Dealler 1991)
	Murex C. albicans	98.3%	99.0%	100%	Germ Tube	(Crist et al. 1995)
	Albicans-Sure (Clinical Standards Labs)	98.7%	99.0%	100%	Germ Tube	(Crist et al. 1995)
	Bacti-Card Candida (Remel)	99.0%	99.0%	100%	Germ Tube	(Crist et al. 1995)
ALL YEASTS	Updated Vitek Yeast Biochem Card	89.7%†			API 20 C	(Fenn et al. 1994; Dooley et al. 1994)
	Updated Vitek Yeast Database	97.2%			API 20 C	(El-Zaatari et al. 1990)
	Microring YT (Medwire/Equip)	52.8%			API 20 C	(Shankland et al. 1990)
	MicroScan (Baxter) Updated	92.0%			API 20 C	(Land et al. 1991)
	MicroScan (Baxter) Updated	96.6%			API 20 C + Corn meal Agar	(St. Germain and Beauchesne 1991)
	RapID Yeast Plus System (Innovative Diagnostics)	95.5%			API 20 C + nitrate + morphology	(Marler and Enriquez 1995)

*See addendum to book for company locations.
†93.0% Common yeasts

ASCOSPORE PRODUCTION

Medium Preparation
Wickerham's malt extract agar:

Malt extract (Difco, BBL)	20 g
Agar	12 g
Distilled water	400 mL

1. For the commercial medium, follow the manufacturer's directions regarding reconstitution. Go to number 3.
2. For homemade malt extract agar, mix the agar and water in a flask on a magnetic stirrer, bring to a boil, cool to 50°C, and add the malt extract.
3. Dispense 10 mL aliquots into screw-capped tubes.
4. Autoclave at 15 psi for 15 minutes, slant the tubes so that there is a 1-inch butt, and allow the medium to harden. Refrigerate.

Procedure
1. Lightly inoculate a room temperature agar slant with portions of three to four young colonies to be tested. Make sure the yeast has been streaked for purity first. Also inoculate positive and negative controls.
2. Incubate at room temperature for 3–5 days, make a smear of the organism and controls, air dry, heat fix, and stain with the modified Kinyoun acid-fast stain (see Color Plate 52).

CHART 5–3. YEAST REACTION PATTERNS

	Assimilations														Fermentations							
	Dextrose	Maltose	Sucrose	Lactose	Galactose	Cellobiose	Raffinose	Inositol	Xylose	Trehalose	Melibiose	Dulcitol	KNO_3	Urease	Dextrose	Maltose	Sucrose	Lactose	Galactose	Trehalose	Growth at 37°C	Pellicle in malt extract broth
Blastoschizomyces capitatum	+	–	–	–	–	–	–	–	–	–	–	–	–	–	–	–	–	–	–	–	+	Wrinkled pellicle; may be submerged
Candida albicans	+	+	+	–	+	–	–	–	+	+	–	–	–	–	G	G	–	–	G	G	+	–
Candida guilliermondii	+	+	+	–	+	+	+	–	+	+	+	+	–	–	G	–	G	–	G*	G	+	–
Candida krusei	+	–	–	–	+	–	–	–	–	–	–	–	–	+*	G	–	–	–	–	–	+	+
Candida parapsilosis	+	+	+	–	+	–	–	–	+	+	–	–	–	–	G*	–	–	–	G*	–*	+*	+
Candida pseudotropicalis	+	–	+	+	+	+	+	–	+	–	–	–	–	–	G	–	G	G	G	–	+	–
Candida tropicalis	+	+	+	–	+	+	–	–	+	+	–	–	–	–	G	G	G	–	G	G	+	+
Cryptococcus albidus var. *albidus*	+	–*	+	+*	–*	+	–*	+*	+	+*	–*	+*	+	+	–	–	–	–	–	–	–*	–
Cryptococcus albidus var. *diffluens*	+	+	+*	–	–*	+	+	+	+	+	+*	+*	+	+	–	–	–	–	–	–	+	–
Cryptococcus gastricus	+	+	+*	–	+	+	+	+	+	+	+*	+*	+	+	–	–	–	–	–	–	–	–
Cryptococcus laurentii	+	+	+	+*	+	+	+*	+*	+	+	+*	+	–	+	–	–	–	–	–	–	+*	–
Cryptococcus luteolus	+	+	+	–	+	+	+	+	+	+	–	+	–	+	–	–	–	–	–	–	–	–
Cryptococcus neoformans	+	+	+	–	+*	–*	+*	+	+	+*	–	+	–	+	–	–	–	–	–	–	+*	–
Cryptococcus terreus	+	–*	–*	–*	–	+	–	–*	+	+*	+	–*	+	+	–	–	–	–	–	–	–*	–
Cryptococcus uniguttulatus	+	+	+	–	–	+	–*	+	+	+*	–	–*	–	+	–	–	–	–	–	–	–	–
Geotrichum candidum	+	–	–	+	+	+	–	–	+	–	–	–	–	–	–	–	–	–	–	–	–*	Pellicle or white islets
Rhodotorula glutinis	+	+	+	–	+	–*	+	–	+*	+	–	–	+	+	–	–	–	–	–	–	+	–
Rhodotorula rubra	+	+	+	–	+*	–	+	–	+	+	–	–	–	+	–	–	–	–	–	–	+*	–
Saccharomyces cerevisiae	+	+*	+	–	+	–	+*	–	–	+*	+*	+*	–	–	G	G	G	–	G	G*	+*	–
Torulopsis candida	+	+	+	+*	+	+	+	–	+*	+	–	+	–	–	G	G	G	–	G	G	+	–
Torulopsis glabrata	+	–	–	–	–	–	–	–	–	+	–	–	–	–	G	–	–	–	–	G	+	+
Trichosporon beigelii (cutaneum)	+	+	+	+	+	+	+*	+*	+	+*	+*	+*	–	+*	–	–	–	–	–	–	+*	Pellicle or ring; blastoconidia seen
Trichosporon penicillatum	+	–	–	–	+	–	–	–	+	+	–	–	–	–	–	–	–	–	–	–	+	White wrinkled pellicle
Trichosporon pullulans	+	+	+	+*	+	+	+*	+	+*	+	+*	–	+	+	–	–	–	–	–	–	+*	Pellicle or ring with islets

+ = Positive   – = Negative   * = Strain variation   G = Gas produced, i.e., fermentation

(Adapted from Warren, NG and Hazen, KC: *Candida*, *Cryptococcus*, and other yeasts of medical importance. In Manual of Clinical Microbiology, ed 6. American Society for Microbiology, Washington, DC, 1995; also adapted from API 20C yeast package insert.)

STUDY QUESTIONS

Circle T if the statement is true and F if the statement is false.

1. T F   All *Candida albicans* produce germ tubes and chlamydospores.

2. T F   A germ tube is constricted at its point of attachment to the mother cell.

For numbers 3 through 6, write the letter(s) of the tests that are most helpful in identifying each of the fungi below.

   A. Corn meal-Tween 80

   B. Germ tube

   C. Malt extract broth

   D. Biochemicals

   E. Ascospore production

   F. Pigment production on caffeic acid agar

   G. Capsules on India ink mount

3. ＿＿＿ *Cryptococcus neoformans*

4. ＿＿＿ *Trichosporon* sp.

5. ＿＿＿ *Saccharomyces* sp.

6. ＿＿＿ *Candida parapsilosis*

7. See Color Plate 56. This yeast is grown on Emmon's agar. On corn meal-Tween 80 agar, only blastoconidia are observed. What is the genus of the organism?

8. See Figure 5–12. This corn meal-Tween 80 microscopic morphology is characteristic of the fungus (genus and species) ＿＿＿＿＿＿＿＿＿＿＿＿＿＿＿＿＿. Note: There are no blastoconidia.

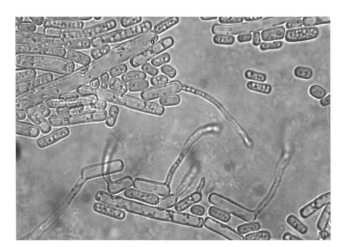

Figure 5–12. Study question demonstration, CM-T80 agar (magnification ×450).

STOP HERE UNTIL YOU HAVE COMPLETED THE QUESTIONS.

Look up the answers in the back of the book. If you missed more than three of them, go back and repeat this section. Correctly complete any missed questions before proceeding.

YEAST DISEASES

CANDIDIASIS Candidiasis (candidosis, moniliasis) is primarily caused by *C. albicans,* although other *Candida* species are becoming increasingly important as disease agents. *C. albicans* exists as normal flora in the throat, vulvovaginal area, skin, and stool. If a patient is immunocompromised, with lowered resistance caused by AIDS, malignancy, lupus erythematosis, diabetes mellitus, tuberculosis, or treatment with steroids or cytotoxic drugs, the yeasts may proliferate and cause an autoinfection. Likewise, if something upsets the balance of bacteria that normally keep yeasts in check, such as prolonged antibiotic therapy, yeasts can proliferate.

Candidiasis in HIV patients. In patients with human immunodeficiency virus (HIV) infection, candidal disease is primarily mucosal. Virtually all patients develop oropharyngeal candidiasis (thrush), which represents intense colonization. However, 80% progress to retrosternal odynophagia (pain on swallowing) typical of yeast esophagitis infection. An endoscopic procedure may be required to explore and to biopsy these lesions, since herpes and cytomegalovirus may produce similar lesions. Vulvovaginal candidiasis is frequent and recurrent. Interestingly, cutaneous infection and disseminated disease are rare.

Once mucosal candidal disease is persistently noted, most physicians would suggest oral antiyeast therapy (fluconazole—see Module 2, Antifungals) prophylactically for the remainder of the patient's life.

Candidiasis in immunosuppressed (non-HIV) patients. C. albicans is still the most prevalent cause of candidiasis. Some of the more recent reports regarding unusual, and increasingly prevalent, strains of *Candida* other than *C. albicans* follow. *C. tropicalis* is seen in cancer and leukemia patients with prolonged granulocytopenia (Warnock and Richardson 1991). *C. parapsilosis* and *C. zeylanoides* are associated with central catheters inserted for extended periods (Branchini et al. 1994; Pfaller et al. 1991). *C. norvegensis* and *C. tropicalis* are associated with peritoneal dialysis and peritonitis (Nielson et al. 1990). *C. guilliermondii* is associated with intravenous drug abuse. *C. zeylanoides* (Pfaller et al. 1991), *C. utilis* (Bougnoux et al. 1993), *C. parapsilosis* (Branchini et al. 1994), and *C. lusitaniae* (Hadfield et al. 1987) are associated with fungemia in immunocompromised patients. It is disturbing that *C. tropicalis, C. lusitaniae, C. guilliermondii,* and *C. parapsilosis* are becoming resistant to amphotericin B.

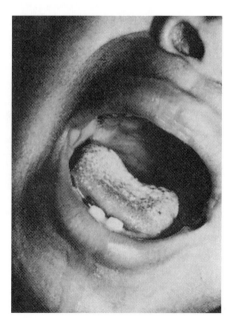

Figure 5–13. Candidiasis of the tongue. (From Rippon: Medical Mycology. WB Saunders, Philadelphia, 1988, with permission.)

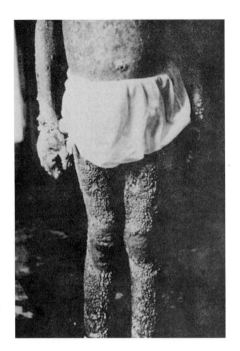

Figure 5–14. Generalized cutaneous candidiasis. (From Rippon: Medical Mycology. WB Saunders, Philadelphia, 1988, with permission.)

Thrush (oral candidiasis, Fig. 5–13) is observed in patients with diabetes mellitus and debilitating diseases such as cancer or tuberculosis. Oral contraceptives and a deficiency of riboflavin also predispose to this overwhelming growth of *C. albicans*. White, creamy patches are seen on the mucous membranes and corners of the mouth. Thrush can progress to esophagitis, especially following chemotherapy.

Yeasts may be carried to the stomach following gastroscopy or surgery, causing gastritis. They can also superinfect preexisting ulcer lesions.

Bronchopulmonary candidiasis is a frequent secondary infection following antibacterial treatment. It can present as a localized or diffuse infiltrate, abscess, fungus ball, or pleurisy (infection of the lung linings). Pulmonary candidal disease versus colonization is difficult to prove unless the organism is seen in tissue.

Cutaneous candidiasis (Fig. 5–14) as a primary infection can be seen in burn patients, but also remember that cutaneous manifestations of disseminated disease (secondary infection) are also possible. Diabetic patients frequently develop localized infection on body areas that are constantly irritated or sweaty (groin, perianal area, under the breasts).

Vulvovaginal candidiasis is usually seen in diabetic patients or those who have finished antibacterial therapy. It may be transmitted sexually, so treatment should begin as soon as possible. Balanitis (inflammation of the glans penis) is most often seen in male diabetics.

In chronic mucocutaneous candidiasis, there is a 50% correlation with an underlying endocrine disorder (adrenal, thyroid), and many times the candidiasis manifests before the endocrine problem.

Candidiasis of the nail (onychomycosis, Fig. 5–15) produces a thickening and hardening of the nail material. Often the skin around the nail is also involved.

Urinary tract infection frequently follows antibiotic therapy or irritation, such as with an indwelling bladder catheter. In noncatheter patients, greater than 10,000 yeasts per milliliter of urine may indicate infection, whereas greater than 100,000 colonies are significant and should be treated. With catheters, *Candida* is usually only colonizing rather than infecting; high colony counts have no meaning, mycelia or blastoconidia are insignificant, and pus cells don't always correlate with infection. Unless the organism is spreading (kidney pain, fever, nausea), most infectious disease specialists do not treat.

Osteoarticular (joint) disease from transient fungemia is seen in heroin addicts and occasionally in the elderly who have had a catheter removed.

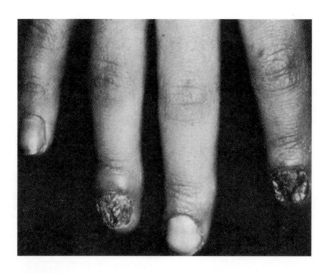

Figure 5–15. Candidal onychomycosis. (From Rippon: Medical Mycology. WB Saunders, Philadelphia, 1988, with permission.)

There exists a new syndrome in heroin addicts, which presents with cutaneous, ocular, and osteoarticular foci of candidiasis. These foci contain 0.5- to 1-cm-sized abscesses resembling bacterial infection, and spontaneously resolve in 3 to 4 weeks.

Endophthalmitis (infection of the inner eye) caused by *Candida* usually results from hematogenous spread.

Peritonitis may be a consequence of (1) peritoneal dialysis *(C. tropicalis, C. norvegensis)*, (2) gastrointestinal (GI) perforation from peptic ulcer disease, neoplasm, or trauma *(C. albicans),* or (3) contamination during surgery *(C. albicans).*

Fifty percent of candidal endocarditis (infected heart valve) cases are from primary infection, such as valvular heart disease, an artificial valve, central venous catheter, cardiac surgery, intravenous lines for hyperalimentation, and heroin addiction. Another cause of candidal endocarditis is an old, residual bacterial endocarditis lesion as a focus for yeast superinfection. Right-sided endocarditis occurs in heroin addicts, with yeasts from the contaminated drug needle entering the vein and continuing to the right side of the heart. Contaminated central venous catheters also lead to the right heart. Signs and symptoms of endocarditis are prolonged fever, new heart murmur, splenomegaly, Osler's nodes, purpura, chorioretinal candidiasis (infection of the eye's choroid membrane and retina), and possibly acute arterial occlusion. Valve vegetations are large and friable. Serial blood cultures are positive in 75 to 80% of endocarditis patients with natural heart valves, but only 50% with prosthetic valves (Warnock and Richardson 1991).

Meningitis presents similarly to other nonfungal causes. Cerebrospinal fluid contains increased protein, low glucose, and pleocytosis.

Disseminated disease presents with a triad of fever, rash, and muscular tenderness. Other signs and symptoms include chorioretinal lesions, confusion, heart failure with rhythm irregularities, decreased blood pressure, disseminated intravascular coagulation, and suppurative thrombophlebitis (pus and venous inflammation with clot formation). *C. tropicalis* is especially associated with disseminated disease. In immunocompromised patients, blood cultures are positive less than 20% of the time, but skin or muscle biopsies are very useful (Warnock and Richardson 1991).

As can be seen from the above description, *Candida* infection has numerous manifestations, some of them life-threatening. With debilitated, immunocompromised patients, do not wait for culture confirmation if there is a high suspicion of systemic disease; start anti-*Candida* therapy first, usually amphotericin B or one of the azoles (see Module 2).

CRYPTOCOCCOSIS Cryptococcosis is caused by *Cryptococcus neoformans var. neoformans* (serotypes A and D) and *Cryptococcus neoformans var. gattii* (serotypes B and C). Cryptococcosis in AIDS patients is associated with the *neoformans* variety. These yeasts are usually isolated from pigeon and other bird droppings, although the birds themselves are not infected. The yeasts are also seen elsewhere in nature: fruits, milk, plants, and feces of normal humans. They are usually inhaled and produce a mild, often subclinical primary pulmonary infection. In fact,

20% of pigeon breeders with no history of infection carry cryptococcal antibody, and patients with chronic lung diseases, such as bronchitis and bronchiectasis, can be asymptomatic carriers. Symptomatic disease manifests as cough and fever with single or multiple nodules in the mid- to lower-lung fields on chest radiographs. Many patients have a dense infiltrate in single lung segments. These infiltrates heal spontaneously in immunocompetent patients; only 18% of untreated patients develop dissemination (Warnock and Richardson 1991), with the remainder demonstrating healed or "walled-off" granulomas. However in patients with underlying diseases, such as AIDS, lymphoma/Hodgkin's, collagen vascular disease, sarcoidosis, renal transplantation, systemic steroid therapy, diabetes mellitus, and rarely carcinoma/leukemia, the infection disseminates. Thus, always treat a pulmonary infection in immunocompromised patients.

Of disseminated diseases, 40 to 86% of cases are meningitis. In normal patients, meningitis may develop over several weeks or years as granulomas or gelatinous cysts containing *Cryptococcus*. In immunosuppressed patients, symptoms develop over days to weeks. Typically, manifestations resemble those of *Toxoplasma* or HIV encephalopathy and include a dull headache, confusion leading to stupor, nausea and vomiting, stiff neck, ataxia (loss of balance), fever, decreased visual acuity, and possibly papilledema (swelling of the optic nerve). Hydrocephalus (fluid accumulation in the brain) is common. Cerebrospinal fluid (CSF) is clear with increased protein, decreased glucose, and usually lymphocyte predominance, but occasionally polymorphonuclear cell predominance. Dissemination involves hepatosplenic infection, osteomyelitis (Gurevitz et al. 1994), subcutaneous disease, and multiple skin nodules with central umbilications similar to molluscum contagiosum. *Cryptococcus* has even been reported to cause prostatitis. Relapses after apparently successful therapy are common, with average survival of AIDS patients after the *Cryptococcus* diagnosis being only 6 months.

Ten to fifteen percent of cryptococcosis is of the cutaneous form. Make certain that it is primary disease rather than a manifestation of disseminated disease.

In tissue, although the standard hematoxylin and eosin (H&E) stain will show non-staining capsules around the yeasts (see Color Plate 57), the mucicarmine stain will make the cryptococcal capsule stand out as a bright rose color, making it much more apparent. This is important if there are only a few organisms in the entire tissue.

Therapy for cryptococcosis is amphotericin B or one of the azoles (see Module 2).

DISEASES CAUSED BY *GEOTRICHUM CANDIDUM*

Geotrichum candidum is seen as a contaminant in soil, cottage cheese, milk, decaying food, tomatoes, and as normal human flora in the mouth, skin, and stool. It rarely produces infection except in debilitated people. Oral infection is characterized by white patches that resemble oral candidiasis, while intestinal disease results in colitis and bloody stools. Bronchial manifestations are the most common form of *G. candidum* infection; the chronic cough and the mucoid, bloody sputum simulate tuberculosis. Vaginal infections, which must be differentiated from candidiasis, have been reported. Rarely, systemic disease, with organisms isolated from blood, has been observed. Other miscellaneous sites include tumefaction in the hand and skin lesions.

In the laboratory, direct mounts reveal fragmenting hyphae with unalternating rectangular arthroconidia possessing rounded ends. *G. candidum* must be distinguished from *Coccidioides immitis*, which usually exhibits alternating arthroconidia. In cultures of throat, stool, sputum, and vaginal specimens, many colonies must be repeatedly isolated before *G. candidum* is considered the etiologic agent of infection. Any organisms recovered from blood are clinically significant.

DISEASES CAUSED BY *TORULOPSIS GLABRATA*

Torulopsis glabrata is isolated from soil and is normal human flora in the oral cavity, urogenital area, and gastrointestinal tract. It is an opportunistic pathogen, usually eliciting disease in debilitated patients. The lungs and kidneys are primarily affected, although the fungus can disseminate through the blood to the rest of the body, causing fungemia and septic shock. A case of congenital transfer has been reported.

In the laboratory, lung tissue may show budding yeast cells inside macrophages similar to *Histoplasma capsulatum*. However, *T. glabrata* has no mold phase, and the isthmus between the budding yeast cells is wider than in *Histoplasma*. Many organisms may be observed in sputum during a lung infection. On urine cultures, 100,000 *T. glabrata* colonies per milliliter of urine are significant, but less than this may also be significant, depending on the patient's clinical condition. Any organisms from blood or spinal fluid are important.

FINAL EXAM   **For questions 1 to 4, refer to the following case study:**

A 45-year-old pigeon breeder, who recently received a renal transplant (and thus was on immunosuppressive steroids), complained to his physician of headache, dizziness, blurred vision, and a stiff neck. Specimens of purulent cerebrospinal fluid were sent to your microbiology laboratory. A carefully examined Gram stain of the CSF sediment was negative; however, on brain heart infusion agar with blood at 30°C, a white, mucoid yeast rapidly grew. The organism was inhibited on brain heart infusion agar with blood, gentamicin, cyclohexamide and chloramphenicol.

1. Which disease do you suspect? Circle the letter of the correct answer.

    A. Candidiasis

    B. No disease — organism was a laboratory contaminant

    C. Histoplasmosis

    D. Cryptococcosis

    E. Coccidioidomycosis

2. Give three reasons for choosing your answer to number 1.

3. If the yeast was significant, why was it not observed on the CSF Gram stain?

4. If your answer to number 1 was not B, what three tests would you perform to speciate the yeast?

5. On a urine bacteriology culture blood agar plate at 24 hours, over 100,000 small, white colonies are observed. They are catalase positive and a slide coagulase test is negative. Your next step is to (circle the letter of the correct answer):

    A. Report over 100,000 *Staphylococcus epidermidis*/mL of urine

    B. Perform a Gram stain

    C. Inoculate a gram-positive urine antibiotic susceptibility battery

    D. Set up a tube coagulase test

    E. Ask for a repeat culture

6. Circle the letter of the correct answer. *Torulopsis glabrata* may be normal flora of:

    A. Stool

    B. Vagina

    C. Throat

    D. All of the above

    E. A and C

STOP HERE UNTIL YOU HAVE COMPLETED THE QUESTIONS.

Look up the answers in the back of the book. If you missed more than one, go back and repeat this module.

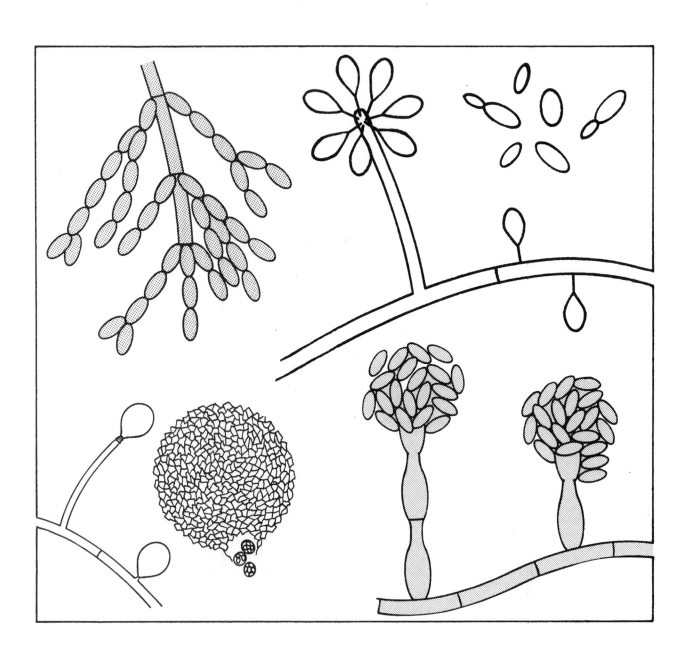

Organisms Causing Subcutaneous Mycoses

PREREQUISITES

The learner must possess a good background knowledge in clinical microbiology and must have finished Module 1, Basics of Mycology, and Module 2, Laboratory Procedures for Fungal Culture and Isolation.

BEHAVIORAL OBJECTIVES

Upon completion of this module, the learner should be able to:

1 Describe the dots and granules from chromoblastomycosis, eumycotic mycetoma, actinomycotic mycetoma, and actinomycosis. Include granule colors, microscopic appearance, causative organisms, and ways to distinguish them from bacterial granules.

2 From culture, microscopic characteristics, and mycosis elicited, recognize the following:

Cladosporium carrionii	*Phialophora verrucosa*
Cladosporium trichoides	*Wangiella dermatitidis*
Exophiala jeanselmei	*Scedosporium apiospermum*
Fonsecaea compacta	*Scedosporium prolificans*
Fonsecaea pedrosoi	*Sporothrix schenckii* ·

3 Differentiate the black yeasts *Exophiala* and *Wangiella* by cultural, microscopic, physiologic, and clinical means.

4 Distinguish between the similar-appearing molds *Cladosporium carrionii* and *Cladosporium trichoides*.

5 Compare and contrast microscopic attributes of *Fonsecaea pedrosoi* and *Fonsecaea compacta*.

6 Discriminate between *Sporothrix schenckii* and the similar-appearing opportunist *Acremonium* sp.

7 Define, identify, or discuss the significance of:

Sclerotic bodies	Two phases of *Sporothrix schenckii*
Cigar bodies	Actinomycete
Daisy head	
Two stages of *Scedosporium* apiospermum	

8 Compare and contrast oxygen requirements, acid-fastness, macro- and microscopic appearance, and odor of the following:
Nocardia sp.
Streptomyces sp.
Group IV Mycobacteria
Actinomyces sp.

9 Briefly describe four physiologic procedures for aerobic actinomycete identification. Include a description of positive and negative results.

10 Concerning anaerobic actinomycetes, list preliminary identification procedures and results recommended prior to sending the organism to a reference laboratory.

11 Briefly describe chromoblastomycosis, phaeohyphomycosis, mycetoma, nocardiosis, actinomycosis, and sporotrichosis, including causative organisms, "dot" or granule characteristics, and mode of transmission.

CONTENT OUTLINE

I. Introduction
II. Molds
  A. Dematiaceous molds
    1. Branching chains of conidia
      a. *Cladosporium carrionii*
      b. *Cladosporium trichoides*
    2. Multiple arrangements of conidia
      a. *Fonsecaea compacta*
      b. *Fonsecaea pedrosoi*
    3. Balls of conidia
      a. *Phialophora verrucosa*
      b. *Exophiala jeanselmei*
      c. *Wangiella dermatitidis*
    4. Chromoblastomycosis
    5. Phaeohyphomycosis
  B. Hyaline molds
    1. *Scedosporium apiospermum*
    2. *Scedosporium prolificans*
    3. *Sporothrix schenckii*
    4. Sporotrichosis
  C. Study questions
III. Funguslike bacteria
  A. Aerobic actinomycetes
    1. *Actinomadura* species
    2. *Nocardia* species
    3. *Nocardiopsis* species
    4. *Streptomyces* species
    5. Tests for aerobic actinomycetes
    6. Nocardiosis
    7. Mycetoma
  B. Mycobacteria
  C. Anaerobic actinomycetes
    1. Actinomycosis
IV. Final exam

FOLLOW-UP ACTIVITIES

1 Students may perform the modified Kinyoun acid-fast stain on *Nocardia* sp. and *Mycobacterium fortuitum,* and compare microscopic features.

2 Students may observe colonies and slide culture preparations of fungi that produce subcutaneous mycoses.

3 Students may convert *Sporothrix schenckii* from the mold to yeast phase.

REFERENCES

Adair, JC, et al: Peritonsillar abscess caused by *Nocardia asteroides*. J Clin Microbiol 25:2214, 1987.

Alvarez, M, et al: Nosocomial outbreak caused by *Scedosporium prolificans (inflatum)*: four fatal cases in leukemic patients. J Clin Microbiol 33:3290, 1995.

Baron, EJ, et al: Processing clinical specimens for anaerobic bacteria: isolation and identification procedures. In Bailey and Scott's Diagnostic Microbiology, ed 9. Mosby-Year Book, St. Louis, 1994.

Baron, EJ, et al: Anaerobic gram-positive bacilli. In Bailey and Scott's Diagnostic Microbiology, ed 9. Mosby-Year Book, St. Louis, 1994.

Beneke, ES and Rogers, AL: Medical Mycology Manual, ed 4. Burgess Publishing Co., Minneapolis, 1980.

Biehle, JR, et al: Novel method for rapid identification of *Nocardia* species by detection of preformed enzymes. J Clin Microbiol 34:103, 1996.

Boiron, P, et al: Urease negative *Nocardia asteroides* causing cutaneous nocardiosis. J Clin Microbiol 28:801, 1990.

Boquest, AL and Tosolini, FA: Letter: Isolation of *Nocardia asteroides* on buffered charcoal-yeast extract agar. J Clin Microbiol 31:1400, 1993.

Bryan, CS: *Petriellidium boydii* infection of the sphenoid sinus. Am J Clin Pathol 74:846, 1980.

Dixon, D: Isolation and characterization of *Sporothrix schenckii* from clinical and environmental sources associated with the largest US epidemic of sporotrichosis. J Clin Microbiol 29:1106, 1991.

Dobson, SRM and Edwards, MS: Extensive *Actinomyces naeslundii* infection in a child. J Clin Microbiol 25:1327, 1987.

Espinel-Ingroff, A, et al: Evaluation of proteolytic activity to differentiate some dematiaceous fungi. J Clin Microbiol 26:301, 1988.

Espinel-Ingroff, A, et al: Evaluation of the API 20C yeast identification system for the differentiation of some dematiaceous fungi. J Clin Microbiol 27:2565, 1989.

Fahal, AH, et al: A preliminary study on the ultrastructure of *Actinomadura pelletieri* and its host tissue reaction. J Med Vet Mycol 32:343, 1994.

Flores, M and Desmond, E: Opacification of middle-brook agar as an aid in identification of *Nocardia farcinica*. J Clin Microbiol 31:3040, 1993.

Hillier, SL and Moncla, BJ: *Peptostreptococcus, Propionibacterium, Eubacterium,* and other non-sporeforming anaerobic gram-positive bacteria. In Murray, PR, et al (eds): Manual of Clinical Microbiology, ed 6. American Society for Microbiology Washington, DC, 1995.

Hironaga, M, et al: Annellated conidiogenous cells in *Exophiala dermatitidis:* Agent of phaeohyphomycosis. Mycologia 73:1181, 1981.

Hollick, GE: Nocardiosis. J Med Technol 1:267, 1984.

Kerr, E, et al: Isolation of *N. asteroides* from respiratory specimens by using selective buffered charcoal-yeast extract agar. J Clin Microbiol 30:1320, 1992.

Kwon-Chung, KJ and Bennett, JE: Medical Mycology, Lea & Febiger, Philadelphia, 1992.

Larone, DH: Medically Important Fungi, ed 3. ASM Press, Washington, DC, 1995.

Larone, DH: Medically Important Fungi. ASM Press, Washington, DC, 1976.

Lennon, PA, et al: Ribosomal DNA internal transcribed spacer analysis supports synonomy of *Scedosporium inflatum* and *Lomentospora prolificans.* J Clin Microbiol 32:2413, 1994.

Luff, RD, et al: Pelvic actinomycosis and the intrauterine contraceptive device: A cyto-histomorphologic study. Am J Clin Pathol 69:581, 1978.

McGinnis, MR: Chromoblastomycosis and phaeohyphomycosis: New concepts, diagnosis, and mycology. J Am Acad Dermatol 8:1, 1983.

Miller, PH, et al: Evaluation of API An-IDENT and RapID ANA II Systems for Identification of *Actinomyces* species from clinical specimens. J Clin Microbiol 33:329, 1995.

Mishra, SK, et al: Identification of nocardiae and streptomycetes of medical importance. J Clin Microbiol 11:728, 1980.

Murray, PR, et al: Effect of decontamination procedures on recovery of *Nocardia* spp. J Clin Microbiol 25:2010, 1987.

Nishimura, K and Miyaji, M: Studies on a saprophyte of *Exophiala dermatitidis* isolated from a humidifier. Mycopathologia 77:173, 1982.

Nolte, FS: Letter: Use of selective buffered charcoal-yeast extract medium for isolation of nocardiae from mixed cultures. J Clin Microbiol 31:2554, 1993.

Paul, C, et al: Chromoblastomycosis with malignant transformation and cutaneous-synovial secondary localization. J Med Vet Mycol 29:313, 1991.

Rippon, JW and Kathuria, SK: *Actinomyces meyeri* presenting as an asymptomatic lung mass. Mycopathologia 84:187, 1984.

Salkin, IF, et al: *Scedosporium inflatum,* an emerging pathogen. J Clin Microbiol 26:498, 1988.

Sanchez-Sousa, A, et al: *Pseudallescheria boydii* genitourinary infection during bladder catheterization in a leukaemic patient. J Med Vet Mycol 30:79, 1992.

Shawar, R, et al: Cultivation of *Nocardia* spp. on chemically defined media for selective recovery of isolates from clinical specimens. J Clin Microbiol 28:508, 1990.

Standard, PG, et al: Exoantigen test for the rapid identification of *Exophiala spinifera.* J Med Vet Mycol 29:273, 1991.

Staneck, JL, et al: Infection of bone by *Mycobacterium fortuitum* masquerading as *Nocardia asteroides.* Am J Clin Pathol 76:216, 1981.

Steadham, JE, et al: Use of carbohydrate and nitrate assimilations in the identification of dematiaceous fungi. Diagn Microbiol Infect Dis 5:71, 1986.

Venugopal, PV, et al: Antimycotic susceptibility testing of agents of black grain eumycetoma. J Med Vet Mycol 31:161, 1993.

Wallace, R, et al: Clinical and laboratory features of *Nocardia nova.* J Clin Microbiol 29:2407, 1991.

INTRODUCTION

Subcutaneous mycoses may develop when the skin is punctured or abraded with thorns or other vegetation contaminated with fungi that live in the soil. The organisms establish themselves in the skin and produce a localized infection in the surrounding underlying tissue and lymph nodes. Rarely does the infection disseminate. Subcutaneous lesions are characterized by chronic, nonhealing, hard, lumpy, crusted, ulcerated areas which periodically exude fluid. The extremities, especially the feet, are often involved, since they come into more frequent contact with thorns and other vegetative structures. Although subcutaneous mycoses are most common in the tropics, they are found worldwide.

In addition to higher fungi, the funguslike bacteria are covered in this module. In primary infections, the latter may produce disease manifestations other than subcutaneous mycoses. For lack of a better place to put them, the nonsubcutaneous diseases caused by funguslike bacteria are included here.

Because the causative organisms of subcutaneous infections are ubiquitous in nature, cultural isolation alone is not significant. Tissue invasion must be demonstrated using potassium hydroxide (KOH) and histopathology preparations.

Specimens are taken from active lesions. If small (0.5 to 2.0 mm), variously colored granules (Fig. 6–1) or black dots are observed on the lesion surface or in oozing fluid, these are also collected. Note the color of the dots and granules, as the color may indicate which organism is producing the infection (Chart 6-1).

In histologic stains or KOH preparations, crushed black dots from chromoblastomycosis appear as thick walled, dark brown, round sclerotic bodies, with a single cell or

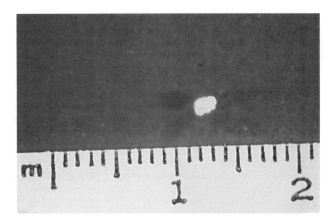

Figure 6–1. White granule. (From Dolan, D, et al: Atlas of Clinical Mycology. ASCP, Washington, DC, 1976, with permission.)

multiple cells formed by cross-walls (Fig. 6–2). Granules from mycetoma exhibit two morphologies: those from higher fungi (**eumycotic mycetoma**) contain pigmented hyphae 2 to 5 μm wide, sometimes accompanied by chlamydoconidia (Fig. 6–3); those from funguslike bacteria (**actinomycotic mycetoma**) contain a center of necrotic debris and peripheral fine, one-micrometer wide, branching, interwoven filaments often surrounded by a gelatinous sheath (Fig. 6–4). The sheath makes the filaments appear club-shaped at the granule edge. Dots and granules are not observed in phaeohyphomycosis or sporotrichosis, and only rarely in nocardiosis.

Specimens are processed as in Module 2. Wash the granules several times in sterile saline to remove contamination before plating. Inoculate specimens to SABHI or BHIB agar with and without antibiotics. If the physician suspects *Actinomyces,* inoculate an anaerobic BHIB plate or a thioglycollate broth.

Organisms causing subcutaneous mycoses are dematiaceous molds, hyaline molds, and funguslike bacteria. Dematiaceous molds may require 3 or 4 weeks to develop, while the light-colored ones grow more rapidly. Funguslike bacteria, which possess dry, glabrous, chalky colonies resembling mycobacteria, vary from rapid to intermediate

CHART 6–1. BLACK DOT AND GRANULE COLORS AND ASSOCIATED DISEASES

Dot/Granule Color and Organisms	Chromoblastomycosis (Black Dots)	Eumycotic Mycetoma (Granules)	Actinomycotic Mycetoma (Granules)	Actinomycosis (Granules)
Brown to black				
Sclerotic bodies (black dots):				
Fonsecaea pedrosoi	X			
Fonsecaea compacta	X			
Phialophora verrucosa	X			
Cladosporium carrionii	X			
Other (granules):				
Exophiala jeanselmei		X		
White to yellow (granules):				
Scedosporium apiospermum		X		
Acremonium falciforme		X		
Nocardiopsis dassonvillei			X	
Nocardia asteroides			X	
Nocardia brasiliensis			X	
Nocardia otitidiscaviarum			X	
Actinomadura madurae			X	
Streptomyces somaliensis			X	
Actinomyces israelii			X	X
Actinomyces bovis			X	X
Arachnia propionica			X	X
Red to pink (granules):				
Actinomadura pelletieri			X	

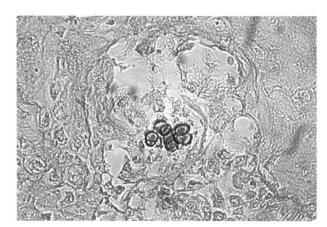

Figure 6–2. Sclerotic bodies in tissue, Gridley stain (magnification ×450).

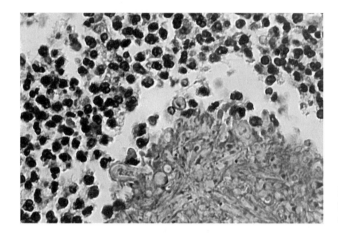

Figure 6–3. Eumycotic granule (bottom half of photo), hematoxylin and eosin stain (magnification ×450).

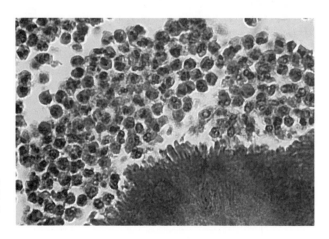

Figure 6–4. Actinomycotic granule with clubbed filaments (bottom half of photo), hematoxylin and eosin stain (magnification ×450).

growing, depending on the species. Mold identification is largely dependent on microscopic morphology. Use of proteolytic activity to differentiate dematiaceous molds recently has been determined to be unreliable and is not recommended. A method for detecting carbohydrate assimilation utilizing the API 20 yeast identification system has been described, but some reactions may be difficult to interpret and the method is not routinely accepted. Thermotolerance studies may be useful to separate some species. Identification of funguslike bacteria incorporates a battery of physiologic tests.

MOLDS

DEMATIACEOUS MOLDS

These organisms may appear as black yeasts at first on SABHI agar, and then later form short, velvety aerial hyphae and conidia. On slide cultures, potato dextrose or corn meal agar is excellent for promoting conidial formation.

The dematiaceous molds are grouped by similar microscopic morphology:

a. Branching chains of conidia
   1. *Cladosporium carrionii*
   2. *Cladosporium trichoides*

b. Multiple arrangements of conidia
   1. *Fonsecaea compacta*
   2. *Fonsecaea pedrosoi*

c. Balls of conidia
   1. *Phialophora verrucosa*
   2. *Exophiala jeanselmei*
   3. *Wangiella dermatitidis*

Important characteristics for each mold are in capital letters. Disease entity, presence of sclerotic bodies or granules, and granule morphology are also important distinguishing features for speciating similar fungi.

Branching Chains of Conidia

Cladosporium carrionii (Figs. 6–5 and 6–6)

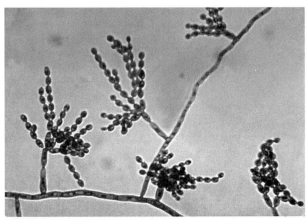

Figure 6–5. *Cladosporium carrionii*, lactophenol cotton blue (LPCB) stain (magnification ×450).

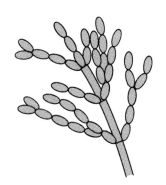

Figure 6–6. *Cladosporium carrionii*.

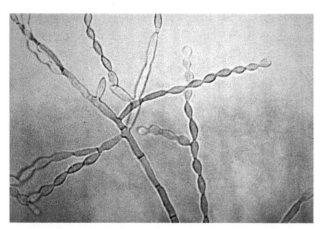

Figure 6–7. *Cladosporium trichoides* (magnification ×690). (From Emmons, CW, et al: Medical Mycology, ed 3. Lea & Febiger, Philadelphia, 1977, with permission.)

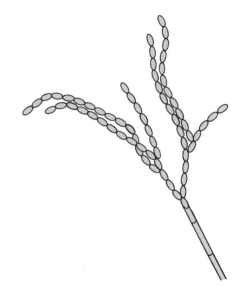

Figure 6–8. *Cladosporium trichoides.*

Culture: On SABHI agar at room temperature, SLOW-GROWING black colonies develop dark velvety mycelium.

Microscopic: The hyphae are dark. Long or short conidiophores support REPEATEDLY BRANCHING SHORT CHAINS OF BLASTOCONIDIA (4.8 to 5.2 μm in diameter). On certain media, phialides with balls of phialoconidia, similar to *Phialophora*, may be observed.

Other comments: C. carrionii DOES NOT GROW AT 42°C and has NO NEUROTROPIC PROPENSITY. *C. carrionii* and *trichoides* are similar morphologically. Growth rate, blastoconidial size, growth temperature, and site of infection should differentiate them. *C. carrionii* does not hydrolyze (liquefy) gelatin.

Pathogenicity: C. carrionii causes chromoblastomycosis.

Cladosporium trichoides (Cladosporium bantianum, Xylohypha bantiana) (Figs. 6–7 and 6–8)

Culture: On SABHI agar at room temperature, a black, compact colony forms MODERATELY RAPIDLY. The reverse is black.

Microscopic: The hyphae are dark. Long or short conidiophores support SPARSELY BRANCHING LONG CHAINS OF BLASTOCONIDIA (7.3 to 7.6 μm in diameter).

Other comments: Considerable controversy exists surrounding the nomenclature of this fungus. *C. trichoides* and *C. bantianum* are now considered to be two separate and morphologically distinct species, both capable of causing subcutaneous and cerebral infections in humans. The recent reclassification of this organism as *Xylohypha bantiana* has been refuted by some mycologists (Kwon-Chung and Bennett, 1992), who found that living cultures of *Xylohypha* sp. did not have dematiaceous vegetative hyphae and had a conidial morphology different from that of *C. trichoides.C. trichoides* GROWS AT 42°C and does not hydrolyze gelatin. In the past, gelatin hydrolysis was considered typical of nonpathogenic *Cladosporium* species, whereas no hydrolysis was considered typical of pathogenic *Cladosporium*; however, this test has proved unreliable.

This organism should always be treated with caution in the laboratory. Work under a microbiological hood and do not set up slide cultures.

Pathogenicity: C. trichoides causes subcutaneous and systemic phaeohyphomycosis and is significant for its tendency to invade neural tissue.

Multiple Arrangements of Conidia

Fonsecaea compacta (Figs. 6–9 and 6–10)

Culture: On SABHI agar at room temperature, a VERY SLOW-GROWING, small black colony develops low, dark velvety mycelium.

Microscopic: The hyphae are dark. PRIMARY BLASTOCONIDIA at the tip of conidiophores each supports one to four SECONDARY CONIDIA, which in turn may produce one to four TERTIARY CONIDIA (Fig. 6–10A). This arrangement culminates in COMPACT CONIDIAL HEADS, while those in similar-appearing *F. pedrosoi* are more loosely organized. Three other types of conidial formation may be less commonly seen: branching chains of blastoconidia as in *Cladosporium* sp. (Fig. 6–10B); one-celled conidia arising opposite each other at the conidiophore tip, the old-named acrotheca sporulation as in *Rhinocladiella* sp. (Fig. 6–10C); and flask-shaped phialides with balls of phialoconidia, as in *Phialophora* sp. (Fig. 6–10D). In the past, identification was based on observation of at least two of the three less common types of conidial arrangements. Now the key morphologic form, the first description above, is employed instead.

Pathogenicity: F. compacta causes chromoblastomycosis.

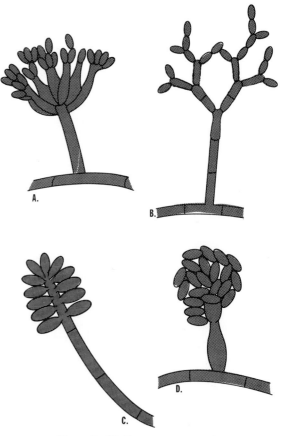

Figure 6–10. *Fonsecaea compacta.*

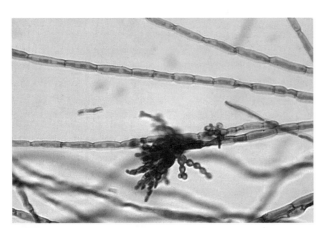

Figure 6–9. *Fonsecaea compacta.* LPCB stain (magnification ×450).

Fonsecaea pedrosoi (Figs. 6–11 and 6–12)

Culture: On SABHI agar at room temperature, a SLOW-GROWING, black colony with low, dark olive to black aerial mycelium is formed (see Color Plate 4).

Microscopic: The hyphae are dark. PRIMARY BLASTOCONIDIA at the tip of the conidiophores each support one to four SECONDARY CONIDIA, which in turn may produce one to four TERTIARY CONIDIA (Fig. 6–12A). This arrangement culminates in LOOSELY ORGANIZED CONIDIAL HEADS, while those of *F. compacta* are more compact. Three other types of conidial formations may be less commonly seen: branching chains of blastoconidia as in *Cladosporium* sp. (Fig. 6–12B); one-celled conidia arising opposite each other at the conidiophore tip, the old-named acrotheca sporulation as in *Rhinocladiella* sp. (Fig. 6–12C); and flask-shaped phialides with balls of phialoconidia, as in *Phialophora* sp. (Fig. 6–12D). In the past, identification was based upon observation of at least two of the three less common types of conidial arrangements. Now the key morphologic form, the first description above, is employed instead.

Pathogenicity: *F. pedrosoi* causes chromoblastomycosis and occasionally systemic phaeohyphomycosis.

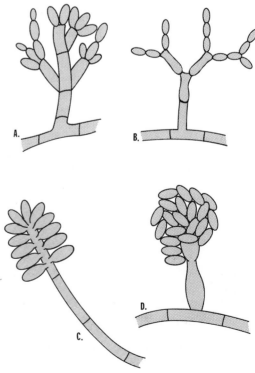

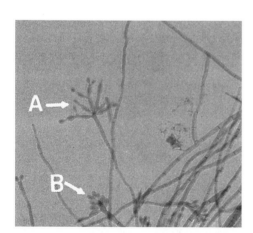

Figure 6–11. *Fonsecaea pedrosoi,* LPCB stain (magnification ×450). Arrow A indicates the key morphologic form; arrow B points to a *Rhinocladiella*-like conidial arrangement.

Figure 6–12. *Fonsecaea pedrosoi.*

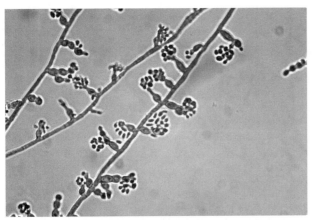

Figure 6–13. *Phialophora verrucosa,* LPCB stain (magnification ×450).

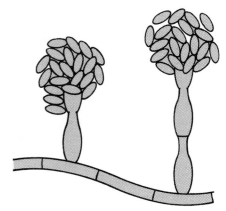

Figure 6–14. *Phialophora verrucosa.*

Balls of Conidia   *Phialophora verrucosa* (Figs. 6–13 and 6–14)

Culture: On SABHI agar at room temperature, a slow-growing black colony with matted dark mycelium is produced (see Color Plate 58).

Microscopic: The hyphae are dark. Flask-shaped PHIALIDES with a distinct CUP-SHAPED COLLARETTE elicit terminal BALLS of oval PHIALOCONIDIA. Phialides may form on the tips of conidiophores or directly off the sides of the hyphae.

Pathogenicity: Phialophora verrucosa causes chromoblastomycosis, subcutaneous phaeohyphomycosis, and rarely keratomycosis.

Exophiala (Phialophora) jeanselmei (Figs. 6–15 and 6–16)

Culture: On SABHI agar at room temperature, a BLACK YEAST forms, which slowly develops dark velvety mycelium (see Color Plate 59).

Microscopic: At first, only dark budding yeasts are observed (Fig. 6–16A). With age, ANNELLIDES on annellophores produce CLUSTERS of oval ANNELLOCONIDIA at the tips (Fig. 6–16B); then the annelloconidia tend to fall down the sides of the stalk (Fig. 6–16b). This second morphology resembles that of *Wangiella* and *Phialophora*. The conidiogenous cell of

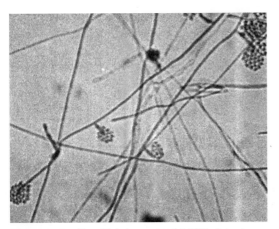

Figure 6–15. *Exophiala jeanselmei,* LPCB stain (magnification ×450).

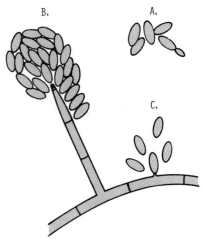

Figure 6–16. *Exophiala jeanselmei.*

Wangiella is tubed like *Exophiala*, but annellations are usually not present. In *Phialophora*, the conidiogenous cell is a vase-shaped phialide. The annellide rings of *Exophiala* may be difficult to discern, but phase contrast and scanning electron microscopy aid greatly in diagnosis. Clusters of conidia may also form off short denticles on the sides of the hyphae (Fig. 6–16C).

Pathogenicity: *E. jeanselmei* causes mycetoma; subcutaneous and systemic phaeohyphomycosis and keratomycosis.

Wangiella (Phialophora, Exophiala) dermatitidis
(Figs. 6–17 and 6–18)

Culture: On SABHI agar at room temperature, colonies are initially shiny BLACK and YEASTY. With time, the periphery develops a dark velvety mycelium.

Microscopic: At first, dark budding yeasts are observed (Fig. 6–18A). With age, a few tubelike PHIALIDES WITHOUT COLLARETTES and usually without annellations* elicit terminal BALLS of CONIDIA (Fig. 6–18B). The conidia tend to fall down the sides of the phialides. Clusters of conidia may also form off short denticles on the sides of the hyphae (Fig. 6–18C). The yeast form remains predominant.

Other comments: *W. dermatitidis* morphologically resembles *E. jeanselmei,* but the former remains more yeastlike. It GROWS AT 42°C (*E. jeanselmei* does not) and is NITRATE NEGATIVE (*E. jeanselmei* is nitrate positive).

Pathogenicity: *W. dermatitidis* causes phaeohyphomycosis.

	NaNO₃ utilization	Max. growth temp. (°C)
C. carrionii	NA	37
C. trichoides	NA	42
E. werneckii	+	42
E. jeanselmei	+	38
W. dermatitidis	−	42

NA = Not Applicable

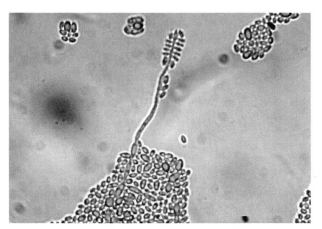

Figure 6–17. *Wangiella dermatitidis,* LPCB stain (magnification ×450).

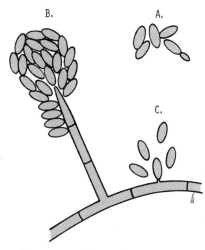

Figure 6–18. *Wangiella dermatitidis.*

*Hironaga et al (1981) and Nishimura and Miyaji (1982) argue that the genus *Wangiella* should be included with *Exophiala,* since annellations are present under electron microscopy. McGinnis (1980) feels that *Wangiella* should stay separate because of its conspicuous yeastlike form and thermotolerance, the inability to observe the annellations with a light microscope, and that phialides rather than annellides are the most distinct, stable, and unique form.

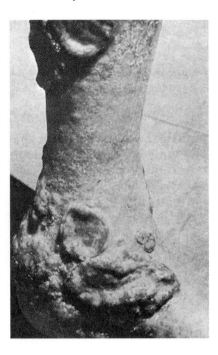

Figure 6–19. Cauliflower lesions of chromoblastomycosis. (From Rippon, J. W.: Medical Mycology. WB Saunders, Philadelphia, 1988, with permission.)

Chromoblastomycosis
(Fig. 6–19)

This infection is almost always limited to the lower extremities, although it has occurred on the hands, face, ear, neck, chest, shoulders, and buttocks. Puncture with contaminated vegetation produces an initial ringwormlike lesion, which very slowly becomes hard, dry, and raised. Many lumps form on top, providing a cauliflower semblance. Usually the eruption is dry, but it may ulcerate. Black dots (sclerotic bodies) are found in the deep part of the lesion. New eruptions spread down the lymphatic drainage, sometimes blocking the lymphatics and producing elephantiasis; bone is not involved. Lesions itch but are basically painless unless secondary bacterial infection ensues.

Up to 15 years may elapse before an entire extremity is involved. In several patients with chronic chromoblastomycosis of more than 10 years' duration, malignant transformation to squamous cell carcinoma has occurred. Fungi causing chromoblastomycosis are all dematiaceous: *F. pedrosoi*, *F. compacta*, *P. verrucosa*, *C. carrionii*, *Rhinocladiella aquaspersa*, and *Cladophialophora ajelloi*.

These agents often are resistant to antifungal therapy, but some cases have responded to treatment with itraconazole. Surgery is often a necessary component of the therapy.

Phaeohyphomycosis
(Chromoblastomy-
cosis in part,
Cladosporiosis)

Phaeohyphomycosis represents a broad spectrum of dematiaceous fungal infections, ranging from superficial involvement to deep-organ disease. In the past, there has been considerable confusion surrounding the terms phaeohyphomycosis and chromoblastomycosis, as the former was designated a special entity of chromoblastomycosis. Now phaeohyphomycosis is described as a separate disease because sclerotic bodies (and also granules) are not evident in tissue; instead, dark yeastlike cells, pseudohyphaelike fungal elements, hyphae, or a combination of these structures appear in the tissue.

The following four categories are useful for classifying phaeohyphomycosis.

A. Superficial—includes black piedra and tinea nigra
B. Cutaneous and corneal—includes dermatomycoses, keratomycosis, and onychomycosis produced by dematiaceous fungi
C. Subcutaneous—usually localized abscesses caused by traumatic implantation. *E. jeanselmei* and *W. dermatitidis* are the most common etiologic agents.

D. Systemic—initial inhalation of the fungus leads to lung infection, which then disseminates to other organs. The brain is often involved, with *C. trichoides* as the most common agent.

Over 70 species of dematiaceous fungi have been recognized as etiologic agents of phaeohyphomycosis. During the past decade, the number of immunocompromised individuals with organ transplants, Cushing's syndrome, autoimmune disorders, leukemias, and AIDS has increased dramatically. Consequently, the increasing incidence of phaeohyphomycosis is beginning to be recognized as a worldwide health problem.

HYALINE MOLDS

Although the hyaline molds listed below may produce dark-colored colonies and conidia, the hyphae and conidia are usually blue in lactophenol cotton blue mounts. Some common light-colored organisms causing subcutaneous disease follow, with key identifying features capitalized.

Scedosporium (Monosporium) apiospermum
(Figs. 6–20, 6–21, and 6–22)

Culture: On SABHI agar at room temperature, a white, fluffy colony develops moderately rapidly, later turning gray with a gray reverse (see Color Plate 60).

Microscopic: In the asexual stage, large, SINGLE or small clustered, oval ANNELLOCONIDIA are TERMINALLY produced on long or short annellophores. The

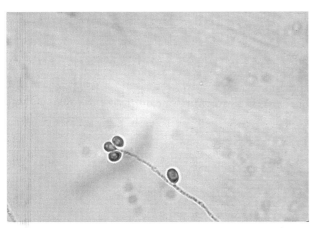

Figure 6–20. Asexual stage, *Scedosporium apiospermum,* LPCB stain (magnification ×450).

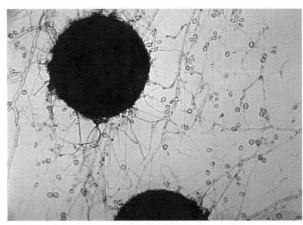

Figure 6–21. Sexual stage cleistothecia, *Pseudallescheria boydii.* In the background is the asexual stage, *Scedosporium apiospermum.* (From Dolan, D, et al: Atlas of Clinical Mycology. ASCP, Washington, DC, 1976, with permission.)

ASEXUAL SEXUAL

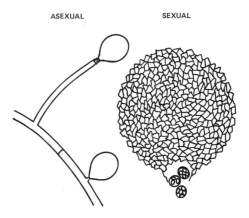

Figure 6–22. (Left) Asexual stage, *Scedosporium apiospermum.* (Right) Sexual stage, *Pseudallescheria boydii.*

annellophores are at the end or on the sides of the hyphae. This asexual morphology is similar to that of the opportunist *Chrysosporium* sp. (Module 3) and the mold phase of the dimorphic fungus *Blastomyces dermatitidis* (Module 7). *Scedosporium* may be differentiated by the diseases it causes and its inability to convert to a yeast phase at 37°C.

Pseudallescheria (Petriellidium, Allescheria) boydii (Figs. 6–21 and 6–22), the sexual stage, may sometimes be observed on potato dextrose or corn meal agar. Large brown CLEISTOTHECIA, 50 to 200 μm in diameter, are seen, which when ruptured disperse ASCI containing 8 light brown, oval ASCOSPORES.

Other comments: With age, the conidia may become slightly dark.

Pathogenicity: S. apiospermum is the most likely agent of mycetoma in the United States. This organism also may cause pulmonary disease, sinusitis, fungus ball, keratomycosis, prostatitis, chronic otomycosis, meningomycosis, and systemic disease.

Scedosporium prolificans (inflatum)
(Figs. 6–23 and 6–24)

Culture: On SABHI agar at room temperature, a white fluffy colony develops moderately rapidly later turning gray with a gray reverse.

Microscopic: Hyaline septate hyphae are seen bearing characteristic annellophores with inflated bases and tapering tips. CLUMPS of oval ANNELLOCONIDIA form at the tips of the annellophores. A sexual stage has not been demonstrated in clinical isolates.

Pathogenicity: Localized infections have been reported including endocarditis, osteomyelitis and arthritis in immunocompetent patients. Disseminated infections have been seen in immunocompromised and neutropenic patients, including fatal nosocomial infections in several leukemic patients. Like *S. apiospermum, S. prolificans* is characteristically resistant to most antifungal agents, but some infections have been treated successfully with ketoconazole or amphotericin B plus flucytosine.

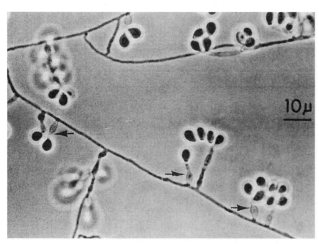

Figure 6–23. *Scedosporium prolificans.* (From Salkin, IF, et al: J Clin Microbiol 1988, with permission.)

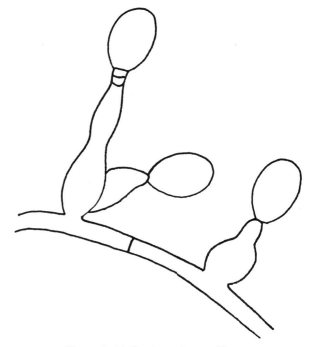

Figure 6–24. *Scedosporium prolificans.*

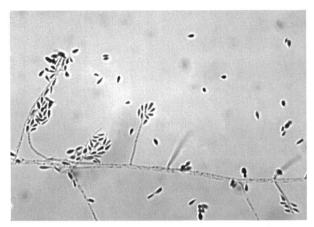

Figure 6–25. Mold phase, *Sporothrix schenckii*, LPCB stain (magnification ×450).

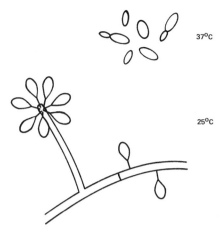

Figure 6–26. Mold and yeast phases, *Sporothrix schenckii.*

Sporothrix schenckii
(Figs. 6–25 and 6–26)

Culture: On SABHI agar at room temperature, this DIMORPHIC fungus forms a cream-colored, wrinkled, leathery colony, which may later turn black. The black color is enhanced on potato dextrose or corn meal agar. The mold phase may resemble the glabrous forms of *Acremonium* sp. (see Module 3), but the latter does not turn black with age. The 37°C yeast phase colonies are soft and white to cream-colored (see Color Plates 61 to 63).

Microscopic: At room temperature, the MOLD appears as small oval hyaline or dematiaceous conidia arranged singly along the hyphae, and as a DAISY HEAD, or flowerette, at the ends of short, unbranched conidiophores. The conidia are attached to the conidiophore by minute hairlike structures, not visible except under oil immersion. The flowerette is not as closely packed as the conidia of the similar-appearing *Acremonium.* Also, the latter cannot be converted to a yeast phase.

    S. schenckii YEASTS are small, elliptical, budding cells resembling cigars; hence the name CIGAR BODIES has been used to describe them (see Color Plate 64). Note that some hyphae may be observed along with the cigar bodies when the fungus is converted in vitro to the yeast phase.

Other comments: The mold is converted to a yeast by subculturing from SABHI agar to brain heart infusion agar, with or without 10% blood, at 37°C in 5% CO_2 for 3 to 5 days. The medium must be kept moist, and one or two rapid serial subcultures may be necessary for yeast formation. Conversion does not need to be complete—in fact, it is difficult in vitro. Any typical yeast cells indicate dimorphism. A viral culture medium of MRC-5 cells (Biowhittaker), also works well for converting the mold to the yeast phase.

Pathogenicity: **S. schenckii** causes sporotrichosis and rarely keratomycosis.

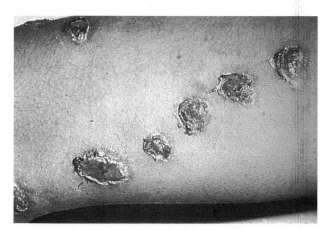

Figure 6–27. Sporotrichosis of arm. (From Dolan, D, et al: Atlas of Clinical Mycology. ASCP, Washington, DC, 1976, with permission.)

SPOROTRICHOSIS
(Fig. 6–27)

This infection usually results from puncture of the skin with contaminated materials such as rose thorns, hay, or wood. Subcutaneous, hard, black, ulcerating lesions are most often seen on the extremities, and they may progress along the lymphatics. Pulmonary sporotrichosis is being observed more frequently, and it must be differentiated from tuberculosis, coccidioidomycosis, histoplasmosis, and sarcoidosis. Rarely, disseminated sporotrichosis may occur.

Epidemics of sporotrichosis have been reported. The largest in the United States occurred in 1988 and involved 84 individuals located in 15 different states. Contact with sphagnum moss grown in Wisconsin was implicated in all cases.

No granules are present in any of the manifestations. Budding yeasts, called cigar bodies, are observed in specimen direct mounts, although the yeasts are not plentiful. Hyphae and conidia are seen on media at room temperature. Conversion of the mold to the yeast phase in vitro is required for identification of the etiologic agent, *S. schenckii*.

The cutaneous form of sporotrichosis has been treated traditionally with oral potassium iodide which remains the most effective form of therapy. Pulmonary or disseminated sporotrichosis requires prolonged treatment with systemic antifungal agents such as amphotericin B and flucytosine, but failures are common. Ketaconazole and itraconazole are less effective, requiring months to years of therapy.

STUDY QUESTIONS

1. Circle the letter of the correct answer.

Cladosporium trichoides and *Cladosporium carrionii* appear similar culturally and microscopically. They may be speciated by all of the following *except*:

A. *C. trichoides* grows at 42°C; *C. carrionii* does not.

B. *C. trichoides* produces sclerotic bodies; *C. carrionii* does not.

C. *C. trichoides* has a predilection for neural tissues; *C. carrionii* does not.

D. *C. trichoides* grows more rapidly than *C. carrionii*.

E. *C. trichoides* exhibits larger blastoconidia than *C. carrionii*.

2. Fill in the chart below, using colonial, microscopic, physiologic, and clinical attributes.

Wangiella dermatitidis
Similarities

1. _____

2. _____

3. _____

Differences

1. _____

2. _____

3. _____

Exophiala jeanselmei
Similarities

1. _____

2. _____

3. _____

Differences

1. _____

2. _____

3. _____

3. Which of the following may demonstrate phialoconidia and cup-shaped collarettes as seen in Figure 6–28? Circle the letter(s) of the correct answer.

A. *Exophiala jeanselmei*

B. *Fonsecaea pedrosoi*

C. *Scedosporium apiospermum*

D. *Fonsecaea compacta*

E. *Wangiella dermatitidis*

F. *Phialophora verrucosa*

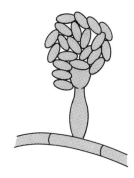

Figure 6–28. Study question demonstration.

4. Circle the correct answer. *Fonsecaea compacta* and *Fonsecaea pedrosoi* may be differentiated from each other in that:

A. *F. pedrosoi* conidial heads are more loosely arranged.

B. Both may exhibit four separate conidial arrangements.

C. Only *F. compacta* produces chromoblastomycosis.

D. *F. compacta* is a rapid grower.

E. *F. pedrosoi* colonies are initially cream-colored and leathery, and later turn black with age.

5. See Figure 6–29. This fungus is the leading cause of eumycotic mycetoma in the U.S. (circle the correct letter):

A. *Cladosporium carrionii*

B. *Sporothrix schenckii*

C. *Scedosporium apiospermum*

D. *Fonsecaea pedrosoi*

E. *Fonsecaea compacta*

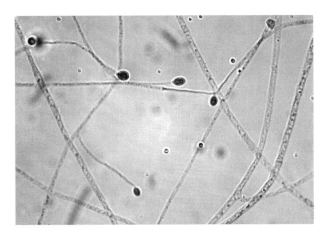

Figure 6–29. Study question demonstration, LPCB stain (magnification ×450).

6. Regarding question 5, what other reproductive structure could you expect to observe?

7. Circle True or False.

    T   F   Cultures of *Scedosporium prolificans* can be identified by observing annellophores with inflated bases and tapering tips bearing oval annelloconidia.

STOP HERE UNTIL YOU HAVE COMPLETED THE QUESTIONS.
Look up the answers in the back of the book. If you missed more than two, go back and repeat the Introduction, Dematiaceous, and Hyaline Fungi sections of this module. Correctly complete any missed questions before proceeding.

FUNGUSLIKE BACTERIA

Funguslike bacteria are microorganisms not classified with the true fungi, but rather with the bacterial subdivision Schizomycota, order Actinomycetales (see Chart 1-2). The term **actinomycete** is used to denote all the Actinomycetales except the family Mycobacteriaceae. Colonies and the microscopic, thin (1 μm in diameter) filaments are typical of bacteria, but the organisms branch, produce conidia, and cause mycoticlike diseases, thus also resembling fungi. The aerobic actinomycetes include the genera *Actinomadura, Nocardia, Nocardiopsis,* and *Streptomyces*.

AEROBIC ACTINOMYCETES
See Chart 6-2.

Actinomadura **species**

Actinomadura sp. are NON-ACID-FAST gram-positive filamentous organisms that grow rapidly on mycobacterial media and other primary isolation media. Growth is enhanced by incubation at 37°C. Colonies are waxy and wrinkled with aerial hyphae that can be seen with a dissecting microscope. Colonies of *A. madurae* are white to pink. This species is a common cause of actinomycotic mycetoma associated with white to yellow granules.

CHART 6–2. SOME PROPERTIES OF AEROBIC FUNGUSLIKE BACTERIA*

	Conidia	Aerial Hyphae	Acid-Fastness	Casein Hydrolysis	Tyrosine Hydrolysis	Xanthine Hydrolysis	Urease	Lysozyme Resistance
Nocardia:								
asteroides	32%+	100%+	61%+	0%+	1%+	0%+	96%+	+
brasiliensis	0	100	78	93	99	0	99	+
otitidiscaviarum	26	100	65	2	14	100	95	+
Actinomadura:								
madurae	15	45	0	98	91	0	0	−
pelletierii	0	24	0	100	100	0	0	−
Nocardiopsis:								
dassonvillei	67	91	0	98	100	100	39	−
Streptomyces:								
somaliensis	14	54	0	100	100	0	0	−
griseus	91	96	0	100	100	97	92	−
sp. (contaminants)			0	+	+	±	±	−
Mycobacterium:								
fortuitum (for								
comparison only)	−	−	+	−	−	−	+	−
Rhodococcus (for								
comparison only)	+	−	+	−	±	−	±	−

*Compiled from Mishra et al (1980) and courtesy of Joseph L. Staneck, Ph.D. and Geoffrey A. Land, Ph.D. (personal communications).

Colonies of *A. pelletierii*, growing on SABHI agar, are pink at first, becoming red with continued growth. When causing actinomycotic mycetoma, bright red granules are observed.

Nocardia species

Nocardia sp. are PARTIALLY ACID-FAST (see box in Module 2 for the modified Kinyoun acid-fast stain). 7H10 and 7H11 agars enhance the acid-fast properties of *Nocardia*, while SABHI, brain heart infusion, and blood agars do not; therefore, transfer suspected isolates to the former media to confirm their staining properties.

Nocardia sp. present in respiratory specimens usually survive mycobacterial concentration procedures and grow rapidly on mycobacterial media. Colonies may be mistaken for mycobacteria: they are chalky, brittle, verrucose, and white to orange* (see Color Plates 9 and 65). However, with *Nocardia*, short aerial hyphae are usually observed under

a dissecting microscope and an EARTHY ODOR, similar to the smell of mud after a rainfall, is exuded. Recently a buffered charcoal yeast extract agar medium (BCYE) used to isolate *Legionella* sp., has been described as a useful medium for primary isolation of *Nocardia asteroides* from respiratory specimens of patients with undiagnosed pulmonary disease. A selective formulation of this medium is especially useful to inhibit normal respiratory flora and facilitate isolation of *N. asteroides*. In addition, media containing paraffin inhibit bacterial overgrowth and allow enhanced recovery of *Nocardia* sp.

Microscopically, branching filaments may fragment into bacillary forms. Tiny CONIDIA may be produced in older cultures, although not in *N. brasiliensis*.

N. asteroides, N. brasiliensis, and *N. otitidiscaviarum* cause nocardiosis and occasionally actinomycotic mycetoma. Tissue granules are not usually observed in the first disease, but they are common in the second.

Nocardiopsis species

Nocardiopsis dassonvillei, which resembles *Actinomadura* sp., is NON-ACID-FAST and grows as a yellow heaped colony on primary isolation media. This species is widespread in the United States, where it may cause actinomycotic mycetoma characterized by cream-colored irregular granules.

---

*Note that isolation media must not contain cycloheximide or chloramphenicol, as these antibiotics suppress funguslike bacteria. Also some strains of *N. asteroides* may be inhibited on SABHI agar. Once purified, aerobic actinomycetes can be cultured on Czapek-Dox agar to enhance colony color and microscopic conidial formation.

Mycobacterium fortuitum can be misdiagnosed as *Nocardia asteroides*:

	N. asteroides	*M. fortuitum*
Acid-fast	+	+
Colonial morphology	variable	variable
Growth at 45°C	±	−
Catalase	+	+
Casein hydrolysis	−	−
Tyrosine	−	−
Xanthine	−	−
Cell wall sugars	Arabinose-galactose	Arabinose-galactose
Gelatin	−	−
DAP in cell wall	meso	meso
INH resistance	+	+

Therapy for these two infections is quite different, with *N. asteroides* requiring sulfa, minocycline, or doxycycline, and *M. fortuitum* requiring antimycobacterial agents. Thus it is imperative for the two organisms to be correctly identified. Perform lipid chromatography: *N. asteroides* contains LCN-A, while *M. fortuitum* does not.

Streptomyces species

Streptomyces sp. are NON-ACID-FAST (although conidia of contaminant strains may be acid-fast) and grow rapidly on most primary isolation media, including mycobacterial inhibitory egg medium. Do not use media with cycloheximide and chloramphenicol. Colonies resemble _Nocardia_ and exude an EARTHY ODOR. Short aerial hyphae are usually observed. Microscopically, branching filaments do not fragment easily, and CONIDIA may be produced with age. _Streptomyces somaliensis_ causes actinomycotic mycetoma, with white to yellow granules. _Streptomyces griseus_ has occasionally been isolated from subcutaneous abscesses and mycetomas. Most _Streptomyces_ sp. are nonpathogenic contaminants.

Since _Nocardia_ and _Streptomyces_ are so similar culturally and microscopically, speciation is primarily dependent on physiologic tests.

Tests for Aerobic Actinomycetes

Nocardia sp. can be distinguished from other aerobic actinomycetes on the basis of their acid-fast staining properties and their lysozyme resistance (i.e., their ability to grow in media containing the enzyme lysozyme). Species of _Actinomadura, Nocardia,_ and _Nocardiopsis_ can be differentiated on the basis of urease production and proteolytic reactions on media containing casein (Fig. 6–30) tyrosine or xanthine (Chart 6-2). _Nocardia_ sp. are usually urease positive; however, urease production is strongly dependent on the type of primary isolation medium used. If a suspected isolate is urease negative, it should be subcultured to a different medium and retested for urease production (Boiron et al. 1990). Quad plates containing each of these three protein media plus urea agar are available commercially (Remel). In addition, _N. asteoroides_ grows at 45°C, whereas _N. brasiliensis_ does not.

N. asteroides is now considered to be a complex of several distinct subspecies. _Nocardia farcinica,_ a characteristically antibiotic-resistant subspecies, has been recognized recently as an etiologic agent of human infections. _N. farcinica_ may be differentiated by its ability to produce a milky-white opacity, within 2 to 10 days, around colonies growing on Middlebrook 7H11 agar (BBL) or 7H10 agar (PML). Recently two identification systems that detect preformed enzymes, the ANA and HNID panels by MicroScan (Dade MicroScan Inc.) accurately identified and differentiated subspecies of _N. asteroides._

If there is still difficulty identifying the funguslike bacterium, it should be sent to a reference laboratory where procedures such as starch hydrolysis, gelatin hydrolysis, sugar assimilations, DAP chromatography, and lipid chromatography can be performed.

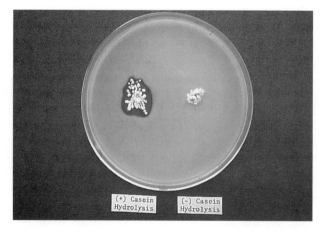

Figure 6–30. Casein hydrolysis. In a positive test, the medium around the colony is clear or hydrolyzed.

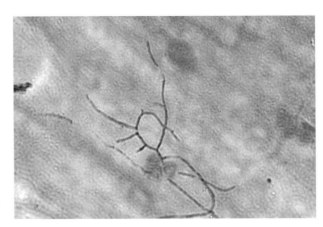

Figure 6–31. *Nocardia* in Gram stain of sputum (magnification ×1000).

Nocardiosis
(Fig. 6–31)

This infection is being seen with increased frequency, especially in patients with cancer or those on corticosteroids. After inhaling the organism, manifestations are initially pulmonary, resembling tuberculosis or bacterial pneumonia. Purulent sputum contains acid-fast branching filaments. Early spread of the disease results in scattered subcutaneous draining abscesses involving the brain and skin, and less frequently, the pleura and heart. Granules are usually not observed. Nocardiosis should be considered whenever the physician suspects tuberculosis, since the clinical manifestations may be similar, the funguslike bacteria are acid-fast, and generalized nocardiosis has a high mortality. Organisms implicated in this disease are *N. asteroides, N. otitidiscavarium,* and rarely, *N. brasiliensis.*

Note that *Nocardia* does not take up the hematoxylin and eosin (H&E) tissue stain; the periodic acid-Schiff and Gridley stains are also not dependable. Thus, diagnosis may be missed in histologic sections. *Nocardia* is effectively demonstrated in the Gomori methenamine silver and Brown and Brenn stains. On sputum smears in the microbiology laboratory, the Gram and modified Kinyoun stains are useful. Sulfonamides are the treatment of choice for nocardiosis.

Mycetoma
(Maduromycosis,
Madura foot)
(Fig. 6–32)

Mycetoma resulting from puncture or abrasion with contaminated material is usually limited to the feet but may be seen on the hands and buttocks. Nodules that periodically exude oily fluid containing white, yellow, red, or black granules slowly progress to involve the entire leg. Infection caused by the higher fungi (eumycotic mycetoma) elic-

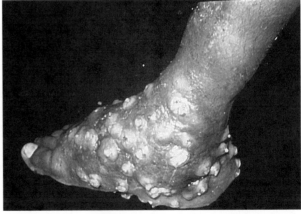

Figure 6–32. Mycetoma of foot. (From Dolan, D, et al: Atlas of Clinical Mycology. ASCP, Washington, DC, 1976, with permission.)

its bored out, punched in lesions, with little pain or bone destruction, while that caused by funguslike bacteria (actinomycotic mycetoma) shows blown-out, conelike lesions, like pimples erupting, with a lot of exudate and painful bone involvement. The extremity becomes greatly enlarged and deformed. As long as 10 to 15 years may ensue before the entire leg is infected. Agents of human eumycotic mycetoma are *Scedosporium apiospermum*, *Acremonium falciforme*, *Acremonium recifei*, *Exophiala jeanselmei*, *Madurella mycetomatis*, and *Madurella grisea*. Organisms producing actinomycotic mycetoma are *Nocardia asteroides*, *Nocardia brasiliensis*, *Nocardia otitidiscavarium*, *Actinomadura madurae*, *Actinomadura pelletierii*, *Streptomyces somaliensis*, *Actinomyces israelii*, and *Actinomyces bovis*.

Eumycotic mycetoma is difficult to treat because many agents are resistant to antifungal agents. Actinomycotic mycetoma can be treated with antibacterial agents: sulfonamide (e.g., sulfamethoxazole-trimethoprim) or dapsone for *Nocardia* sp. and *Streptomyces* sp.; or penicillins for *Actinomyces* sp.

MYCOBACTERIA

Runyon Group IV rapid-growing mycobacteria are not funguslike bacteria, but they are easily confused with the aerobic actinomycetes. It is desirable to learn some distinguishing characteristics of the former in order to rule them out. Mycobacteria are aerobic, growing well on TB media and sometimes on fungal media. Colonies are brittle or smooth, beige to yellow-orange, and no aerial hyphae are produced. An earthy odor is not present. Mycobacteria are acid-fast, even after decolorizing for three minutes. Microscopically, short bacillary filaments rarely branch and no conidia are produced. Physiologic tests give reactions characteristic for each mycobacterial species. These organisms do not cause mycetoma.

ANAEROBIC ACTINOMYCETES
(Figs. 6–33 and 6–34)

Anaerobic actinomycetes are ANAEROBIC, facultatively anaerobic, or microaerophilic; they are not acid-fast in culture and grow in 7 to 10 days. On anaerobic blood agar or BHIB agar at 37°C under an atmosphere of 95% N_2 and 5% CO_2, colonies are small, white, and flat or centrally indented, resembling a MOLAR TOOTH (see Color Plate

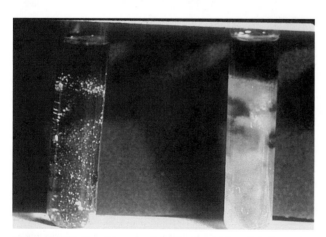

Figure 6–33. Bread crumb and diffuse colonies of *Actinomyces* in thioglycollate broth. (From Jones, JW, et al: Atlas of Medical Mycology. ASCP, Chicago, 1967, with permission.)

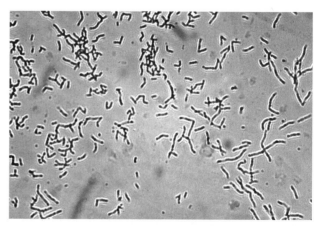

Figure 6–34. Gram stain of *Actinomyces* (magnification ×1000).

66). In thioglycollate broth (Fig. 6–33), pure cultures present a BREAD CRUMB or diffuse appearance. Microscopically, long or short BRANCHING FILAMENTS AND DIPHTHEROID FORMS are observed. On Gram stains of clinical material (Fig. 6–34). *Actinomyces* may appear as gram-positive rods or coccobacilli due to fragmentation, and the organism can be mistaken for diphtheroids. No conidia are produced.

Actinomyces israelii and *naeslundii* are isolated as normal flora from saliva and tonsillar crypts. Sputum may contain anaerobic actinomycetes, reflecting colonization rather than infection; thus, for suspected pulmonary actinomycosis, specimens of choice are lung biopsy, pulmonary needle aspiration, or pleural fluid. *Actinomyces israelii, Actinomyces bovis. Actinomyces naeslundii, Actinomyces meyeri, Actinomyces viscosus. Arachnia propionica,* and *Bifidobacterium dentium (eriksonii)* may cause actinomycosis. The characteristic sulfur-colored granules associated with this disease are produced by some but not all *Actinomyces* sp. and *Arachnia propionica,* while *Bifidobacterium dentium* does not exhibit them. Note that bacteria may form granules resembling those of funguslike bacteria, and the causative organisms must be differentiated physiologically. *A. israelii* and *bovis* may cause actinomycotic mycetoma, with oozing sinuses containing sulfur granules.

Examine streaked anaerobic plates under a dissecting microscope at 48 hours and again at 7 to 10 days to observe the colonial morphology. Perform a Gram stain and inoculate three brain heart infusion slants with an isolated colony of the test organism. Incubate one slant aerobically. After 24 to 48 hours at 37°C, or when there is good colony formation, compare the growth in each tube (see Chart 6-3 for results).

Perform a catalase test by adding 3% H_2O_2 to the brain heart infusion slant with the best growth. Be sure to wait at least 30 minutes after removing the slant from anaerobic incubation before adding H_2O_2. Bubbles indicate a positive test, while absence of bubbles indicates a negative result. Anaerobic diphtheroids, *Propionibacterium* sp., are catalase-positive, and anaerobic actinomycetes are catalase-negative.

At this point, send the organism to a reference laboratory for further identification, or perform nitrate reduction, starch hydrolysis, and mannitol and mannose fermentation tests. Other tests that may be performed as needed are gelatin liquefaction, litmus milk reaction, more sugar fermentations, indole production, and gas-liquid chromatography.

One of the following rapid or automated systems may be used for preliminary identification of *Actinomyces* sp., but conventional biochemical tests are recommended for definitive identification.

Commercial anaerobe identification systems:

API 20A and API An IDENT (bioMerieux, Vitek, Inc.)
Anaerobe-Tek (Remel)
RapID ANA (Innovative Diagnostics, Inc.)
Minitek and Crystal (Becton-Dickinson Microbiology Systems)

Automated systems for anaerobic identification:

MicroScan (Baxter-American MicroScan)
Vitek (bioMerieux, Vitek, Inc.)

Actinomycosis
(Fig. 6–35)

Unlike the other subcutaneous mycoses, actinomycosis has an endogenous origin: the main causative agents are normal anaerobic flora of the mouth. When the oral mucous membranes become injured (e.g., after a tooth extraction), the organisms infect the adjacent face and neck areas, producing swollen, hard, lumpy, draining abscesses (**lumpy jaw**, Fig. 6–35). If the funguslike bacteria are aspirated into the lungs, they produce pulmonary or thoracic actinomycosis characterized by cough, fever, mucopurulent bloody sputum, and multiple draining lung sinuses, which may contain sulfur-colored granules. Pulmonary disease may simulate tuberculosis. If *Actinomyces* sp. are swallowed, they produce abdominal disease with symptoms of appendicitis or carcinoma. Primary pelvic actinomycosis associated with the intrauterine device has been reported. Systemic spread from the jaw, lungs, or gastrointestinal tract may include the skin, kidneys, genital tract, liver, ovaries, bones, joints, and central nervous system. Draining pus contains sulfur-colored granules or masses of gram-positive branching filaments. The prognosis is very good if the disease is diagnosed early. Unfortunately, physicians often do not sus-

CHART 6–3. IDENTIFICATION OF ANAEROBIC ACTINOMYCETES*

	Actinomyces israelii	Actinomyces bovis	Actinomyces naeslundii	Bifidobacterium dentium	Arachnia propionica
Aerobic growth	1+	2+	2+ (best grown in 5% CO_2)	0	1–2+
Anaerobic growth	4+	4+	4+	4+	4+
48-hour colony on BHI agar, anaerobically incubated (examine under microscope)	Spidery, dense mycelial center with lacey border	Circular, granular to smooth; slightly raised center with an entire edge	Resembles A. israelii (spidery form with dense center)	Flat, granular with dense hyphal core	Resembles A. israelii
7–10-day colony on BHI agar (anaerobic)	Raised, rough; lobular; like a molar tooth	Flat to convex; opaque with smooth to pebbly edges	May resemble A. israelii or A. bovis; most often similar to A. bovis	Resembles A. bovis; usually has scalloped edge	Resembles A. bovis; smooth and flat
Growth in thioglycollate broth, 37°C	Discrete, bread crumb colonies without turbidity	Turbidity with dense sediment	Rough colonies or soft diffuse growth; somewhat cloudy	Soft colonies, diffuse growth	Diffuse or turbid growth
Microscopic morphology (all are gram +)	Branching, diphtheroid forms	Diphtheroid forms most usual; branching rarely seen	Branching, diphtheroid forms	Branching, diphtheroid forms	Branching, diphtheroid forms; long branching forms with age
Catalase	0	0	0	0	0
Nitrate reduction	80% +	0	90% +	0	+
Starch hydrolysis	0 or ±	4+	0 or ±	4+	0
Mannitol fermentation	V	0	0	A	±
Mannose fermentation	A	0 or ±	A	A	A
Other test results: Gelatin hydrolysis	0 (occasionally late +)	0	0	0	0
Glucose fermentation	A	A	A	A	A
Xylose fermentation	80% A	0^V	0	A	A
Raffinose fermentation	V	0	80% A	A	A

*Compiled from Larone (1976) and Beneke, ES and Rogers, AL: Medical Mycology Manual, ed 4. Burgess Publishing Co., Minneapolis, 1980.

A = Acid
V = Variable
0 = Negative
+ = Positive
± = Weak reaction

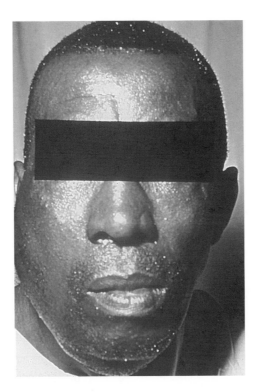

Figure 6–35. Actinomycosis of jaw. (From Dolan, D, et al: Atlas of Clinical Mycology. ASCP, Washington, DC, 1975, with permission.)

pect actinomycosis, and many laboratories do not routinely inoculate anaerobic bacterial media when fungal culture is requested. Organisms causing the disease are *A. israelii, A. bovis, A. naeslundii, A. meyeri, A. viscosus, Bifidobacterium dentium (ericksonii),* and *Arachnia propionica.* Penicillin compounds are the treatment of choice for actinomycosis.

FINAL EXAM   *Place the letter(s) of the genera below in front of the corresponding characteristics.*

    A. *Actinomyces* sp.

    B. *Streptomyces* sp.

    C. *Nocardia* sp.

    D. *Mycobacterium* sp.

1. _____ Acid-fast

2. _____ Anaerobic

3. _____ Earthy odor

4. _____ Conidia

5. _____ Molar tooth appearance on agar

6. Circle true or false.

    T F   Only fungi and funguslike bacteria may produce granules in tissue.

7. Red granules are observed in a foot lesion. Microscopically, the crushed granules contain fine, 1-μm wide, branching filaments radiating out from a center of necrotic material. The patient most likely has (circle the letter of the correct answer):

    A. Chromoblastomycosis

    B. Eumycotic mycetoma

    C. Actinomycotic mycetoma

    D. Actinomycosis

    E. Sporotrichosis

8. *Sporothrix schenckii* resembles *Acremonium,* an opportunist which may cause mycetoma. How may they be differentiated? Describe two ways.

9. Circle the correct letter. Which of the following exhibits polymorphism, in which more than one type of conidial arrangement may be observed?

   A. *Cladosporium carrionii*

   B. *Phialophora verrucosa*

   C. *Fonsecaea pedrosoi*

   D. *Fonsecaea compacta*

   E. A, C, and D

   F. All of the above

10. Match the letter of the organisms with the appropriate test(s) in the list below.

   A. Anaerobic actinomycetes   1. Casein, tyrosine, xanthine

   B. Aerobic actinomycetes   2. Gelatin liquefaction

   C. Both   3. KOH preparation for sclerotic bodies

   D. Neither   4. Catalase, fermentations

Circle true or false:

11. T F Granules are seen in mycetoma caused by *Nocardia*, yet, in nocardiosis, granules are usually not observed.

12. T F Characteristic sulfur-colored granules are usually present in both actinomycosis and mycetoma produced by the same organisms.

13. T F In the past, phaeohyphomycosis was considered a part of chromoblastomycosis. Now the two are separated by the lack of sclerotic bodies in phaeohyphomycosis.

14. Chromoblastomycosis and mycetoma are both slowly-progressing infections which affect the extremities. Describe two ways they may be differentiated.

15. Circle the correct letter.

   The subcutaneous disease with an endogeneous (within self) origin is:

   A. Sporotrichosis

   B. Actinomycosis

   C. Phaeohyphomycosis

   D. Eumycotic mycetoma

   E. Chromoblastomycosis

For the next three questions, refer to this case study.

   A 35-year-old rose gardener noticed a hard, immovable lump under the skin of his index finger but decided to ignore it. A month later, the lump ulcerated to present a black, necrotic appearance, and two more lesions developed further up the wrist and forearm. At this point, he visited his physician. A histologic stain of material from deep in the lesions showed rare elongated yeast cells resembling cigars. On SABHI agar at room temperature, a cream-colored leathery colony grew relatively rapidly, and after 9 days it started to turn black.

16. What disease is suspected and why? Give two reasons.

17. What would you expect to see in microscopic mounts from the SABHI? Circle the letter of the correct answer.

    A. Hyaline cigar bodies

    B. Dematiaceous annellides with terminal conidia

    C. Hyaline daisy head flowerettes of conidia

    D. Single terminal, hyaline conidia

    E. Hyaline, tapering conidiophores with terminal balls of conidia

18. The etiologic agent is ubiquitous in nature. How did the patient probably contract the fungus?

For the next two questions, refer to this case study.

    Black sclerotic bodies were observed on crusty, cauliflowerlike foot lesions of a 30-year-old male Indian patient from South America. Culture of the crushed black dots onto SABHI agar revealed a slow-growing black, velvety colony. Microscopically, there was only the conidial arrangement seen in Figure 6–36.

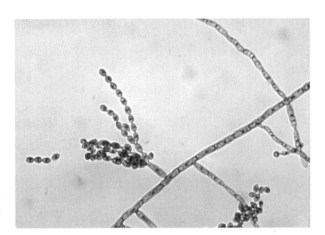

Figure 6–36. Study question demonstration, LPCB stain (magnification ×450).

19. What disease is suspected and why? Give two reasons.

20. The etiologic agent is most likely (circle the letter of the correct answer):

    A. *Cladosporium trichoides*

    B. *Fonsecaea pedrosoi*

    C. *Fonsecaea compacta*

    D. *Exophiala jeanselmei*

    E. *Cladosporium carrionii*

STOP HERE UNTIL YOU HAVE COMPLETED THE QUESTIONS.

Look up the answers in the back of the book. If you missed more than three, go back and repeat this module. Correctly complete any missed questions.

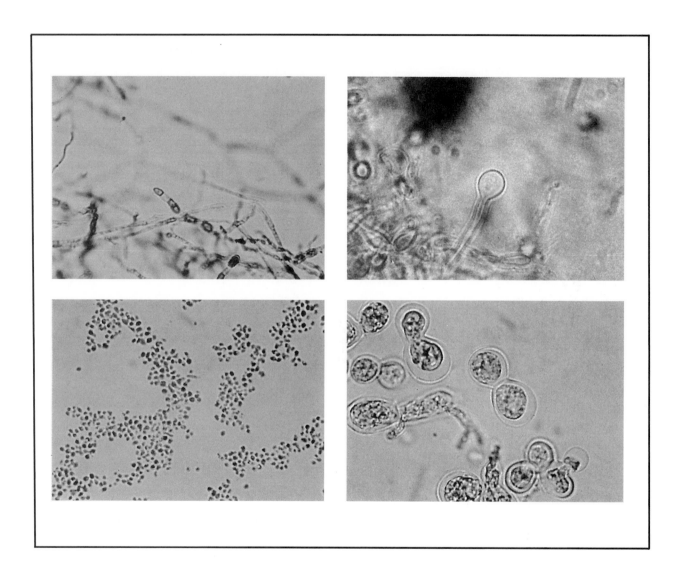

MODULE

7

Organisms Causing Systemic Mycoses

PREREQUISITES

The learner must possess a good background knowledge in clinical microbiology and must have finished Module 1, Basics of Mycology, and Module 2, Laboratory Procedures for Fungal Culture and Isolation.

BEHAVIORAL OBJECTIVES

Upon completion of this module, the learner should be able to:

1 List two properties that *Blastomyces dermatitidis, Paracoccidioides brasiliensis, Histoplasma capsulatum,* and *Coccidioides immitis* all share.

2 Discuss safety precautions to use when working with systemic pathogens.

3 List two reasons why direct mounts are especially useful when working with suspected systemic fungi.

4 From specimen direct mounts, identify characteristic fungal structures associated with the systemic agents in objective number 1.

5 Convert *Blastomyces, Paracoccidioides,* or *Histoplasma* from the mold to yeast phase and discuss special conditions necessary for conversion.

6 Identify from culture, microscopic preparations, and disease descriptions the organisms listed in objective number 1.

7 Differentiate the systemic pathogens from other similar-appearing organisms.

8 Briefly describe blastomycosis, paracoccidioidomycosis, histoplasmosis, and coccidioidomycosis, including any special epidemiologic (geographic) associations, mode of transmission, causative agents, and main types of clinical infection.

CONTENT OUTLINE

FOLLOW-UP ACTIVITIES

1 Students may observe room temperature colonies, 37°C colonies, and tease preparations of fungi that cause systemic mycoses.
2 Students may convert *Blastomyces dermatitidis* from the mold to yeast phase.

REFERENCES

Blotta, MH and Camargo, CP: Immunological response to cell-free antigens of *Paracoccidioides brasiliensis:* Relationship with clinical forms of paracoccidioidomycosis. J Clin Microbiol 31:671, 1993.

Chaturvedi, S, et al: Cottonseed extract vs Pharmamedia for the in-vitro mould-yeast conversion of *Blastomyces dermatitidis.* J Med Vet Mycol 28:139, 1990.

Galgiani, JN, et al: *Coccidioides immitis* in AIDS patients. In Bossche, V (ed): Mycoses in AIDS Patients. Plenum Press, New York, 1990.

Graybill, JR, et al: The major endemic mycoses in the setting of AIDS: clinical manifestations. In Bossche, V (ed): Mycoses in AIDS Patients. Plenum Press, New York, 1990.

Hostetler, JS, et al: Treatment of coccidioidomycosis with SCH 39304. J Med Vet Mycol 32:105, 1994.

Musial, CE, et al: Recovery of *Blastomyces dermatitidis* from blood of a patient with disseminated blastomycosis. J Clin Microbiol 25:1421, 1987.

Rinaldi, MG: Histoplasma in AIDS patients. In Bossche, V (ed): Mycoses in AIDS Patients. Plenum Press, New York, 1990.

San-Blas, G: Paracoccidioidomycosis and its etiologic agent *Paracoccidioides brasiliensis.* J Med Vet Mycol 31:99, 1993.

Smith, MA, et al: An unusual case of coccidioidomycosis. J Clin Microbiol 32:1063, 1994.

INTRODUCTION

In this module, those organisms that classically cause systemic mycoses (i.e., *Blastomyces dermatitidis, Paracoccidioides brasiliensis, Histoplasma capsulatum,* and *Coccidioides immitis*) are described. Recently *Pneumocystis carinii,* which also causes systemic disease, was transferred from parasitic to fungal status. There are numerous, excellent parasitology texts available, which cover *Pneumocystis.*

Systemic fungi typically disseminate throughout the body's organ systems. Note, however, that cutaneous manifestations caused by systemic fungi may cause some confusion. The organisms may have produced infection throughout the body, with secondary spread to the skin. Alternatively, these organisms may be capable of causing a primary cutaneous infection with no evident systemic manifestations. Also, many opportunistic fungi may elicit systemic disease under the proper conditions, for example, in debilitated or immunosuppressed patients. Opportunists were covered in previous modules.

Specimens are collected as described in Module 2. Direct mounts are a must; since the four fungi listed above are the dimorphic and mold phases of all except *Coccidioides* are slow-growing, a rapid preliminary identification is facilitated by observing the tissue phases in direct mounts. The tissue phases (Chart 7-1) can be seen in unstained wet preparations of specimens, for example in sputum, although histology stains such as PAS, GMS, and H&E are more definitive. *Blastomyces* exhibits thick-walled budding yeasts, with a broad base of attachment between the mother and daughter cell. *Coccidioides* spherules are difficult to grow in vitro and thus may be seen only in direct mounts (see Color Plate 67) unless animal studies are performed, which are beyond the scope of most clinical laboratories. Animal studies also require a longer turnaround time than is useful for the physician and patient. In histoplasmosis a Wright stain of infected blood or bone marrow will reveal pseudoencapsulated yeast forms of *Histoplasma capsulatum,* with a narrow isthmus between mother and daughter cells. The yeasts are observed inside reticuloendothelial cells (monocytes and neutrophils). Regular histology stains of various tissues show the same morphology as the Wright stain (see Color Plate 68). Although rare in the United States, *Paracoccidioides* should not be overlooked; multiple thick-walled daughter yeasts bud off a large mother cell (see Color Plate 13).

Unfortunately, organisms may be sparse and overlooked in tissue stains. The long incubation period of these fungi and the need for quick intervention with appropriate

CHART 7-1. MICROSCOPIC MORPHOLOGY OF SYSTEMIC PATHOGENS

Blastomyces dermatitidis	*Paracoccidioides brasiliensis*	*Histoplasma capsulatum*	*Coccidioides immitis*

MOLD PHASE

TISSUE PHASE

antifungal therapy has spawned a new technology. The polymerase chain reaction (PCR) can detect as little as a single strand of fungal DNA in the patient specimen, and restriction enzymes can identify it before the specimen is even placed onto culture media! This technology is still in its infancy, but holds much promise.

Currently, the more established methods involve identifying the organism that was first grown in culture, by exoantigen testing, DNA probe, microscopic morphology, or conversion to the yeast (tissue) phase. Additionally, paired acute and convalescent sera may be tested by several methods to determine if there is a fourfold rise in titer against one of the test antigens. For further information about exoantigen testing, DNA probe, PCR, or serum testing, see Module 2.

SABHI agar or brain heart infusion agar with blood is inoculated with specimen. Antibiotics may be added to the medium to inhibit contaminants. If specimens are respiratory in origin, they must be decontaminated and concentrated (see Module 2) before inoculating the media. Slants are preferred over plates for all systemic fungi, especially *Coccidioides,* because there is less chance for the mold phase to become airborne and infect laboratory personnel. Media are incubated at room temperature for up to 12 weeks.

With the exception of *Coccidioides,* which is an intermediate grower, the other systemic pathogens grow slowly at 25°C, requiring 3 to 6 weeks to form a mature culture. Colonies are initially membranous but later develop white to tan aerial mycelia. Lactophenol tease mounts reveal septate hyphae and conidia or arthroconidia. Do not inoculate slide cultures with suspected systemic molds for safety reasons. Conversion to the tissue phase is the confirmatory identification for dimorphic fungi (box).

Mold forms of systemic organisms are highly infective. Wear mask and gloves while working under a microbiologic hood. It is preferable to put 10% formalin over the culture and leave it overnight before preparing tease mounts, but first transfer some of the colony to media at 25°C and 37°C to maintain viable colonies for further studies.

CONVERSION OF DIMORPHIC FUNGI FROM THE MOLD TO YEAST PHASE

Conversion medium:
Brain heart infusion agar with 10% blood, cottonseed extract (Charturvedi et al. 1990), or Pharmamedia.

Procedure
1. Place a small amount of the test mold on a slant of conversion medium. Keep the surface moist with 0.5 mL sterile distilled water or sterile brain heart infusion broth. Make sure the mold is placed approximately 5 mm above the liquid.
2. Incubate at 37°C for 3 to 5 days. Keep test tube caps loose.
3. Take a portion of the resultant colony which has the most yeastlike consistency and transfer it to a fresh slant of conversion medium, adding moisture as above.
4. Reincubate at 37°C for 3 to 5 days and continue to make serial transfers until the colony grows as a yeast, or until yeast forms are demonstrated microscopically in lactophenol cotton blue tease mounts.
5. Some dimorphic strains, especially those of *Histoplasma,* do not readily convert to a yeast phase. If the fungus does not form a yeast in 14 days, inoculate a fresh slant and send it to a reference laboratory for further identification. *Coccidioides* remains a mold at both 25°C and 37°C and will not produce spherules with this method.

ORGANISMS AND DISEASES

Key identifying features are in capital letters.

BLASTOMYCES DERMATITIDIS
(Figs. 7–1 and 7–2)

Culture: On SABHI agar at room temperature, a yeastlike colony initially develops. With time, the center becomes prickly and later the entire colony is fluffy white or tan (see Color Plate 69).

On brain heart infusion agar with blood at 37°C, colonies are waxy, wrinkled, and cream to tan-colored (see Color Plate 70). Conversion from the mold to yeast phase takes 4 to 5 days.

Microscopic: Tease mounts of the room temperature colony (MOLD phase) show SINGLE smooth-walled, round to oval CONIDIA at the ENDS of short conidiophores or directly on the hyphae. The mold phase may microscopically resemble the opportunist *Chrysosporium* sp. (see Module 3) or the subcutaneous pathogen *Scedosporium apiospermum* (see Module 6). *Blastomyces dermatitidis* may be differentiated by its slow growth rate

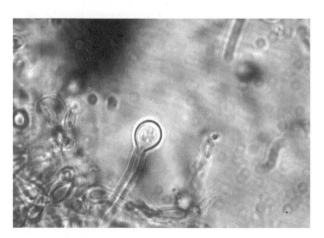

Figure 7–1. Mold phase, *Blastomyces dermatitidis,* lactophenol cotton blue (LPCB) stain (magnification ×1000).

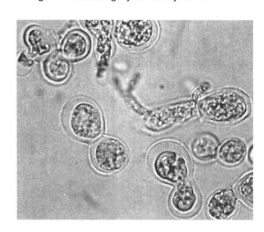

Figure 7–2. Yeast phase, *Blastomyces dermatitidis,* LPCB stain (magnification ×1000).

(*Chrysosporium* = rapid, *Scedosporium* = intermediate) and by its ability to convert to a yeast phase (neither of the others can do this).

The 37°C YEAST phase microscopically appears as large, round, THICK-WALLED, SINGLE-BUDDING yeast cells with a BROAD ISTHMUS where the daughter cell attaches to the mother.

Pathogenicity: B. dermatitidis causes blastomycosis.

BLASTOMYCOSIS (NORTH AMERICAN BLASTOMYCOSIS, GILCHRIST'S DISEASE) (Figs. 7–3 and 7–4)

Blastomycosis, caused by *B. dermatitidis,* is classically observed south of the Ohio River and east of the Mississippi River. There are, however, cases reported from Canada, Latin America, Africa, and elsewhere. *Blastomyces* are thought to be inhaled and they produce a mild chronic respiratory infection, which gradually worsens over weeks or months. Sputum becomes purulent and blood-streaked. The respiratory disease is similar to tuberculosis, coccidioidomycosis, paracoccidioidomycosis, and histoplasmosis; it must be carefully differentiated by cultural and histologic methods. Without treatment the infection usually disseminates to the rest of the body, starting in adjacent subcutaneous tissues. Skin and bone lesions are particularly associated with systemic spread. Skin lesions are ulcerated and crusted or weepy, with small abscesses in the center. The oral and nasal mucosa may be involved. Bone lesions produce pain and loss of function, with the vertebrae and ribs most often affected. In contrast to histoplasmosis and paracoccidioidomycosis, the gastrointestinal tract is rarely infected in blastomycosis. Rarely, the or-

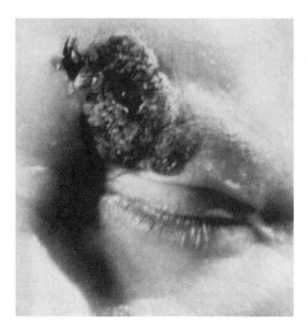

Figure 7–3. Primary cutaneous blastomycosis of eyebrow. (From Beneke, E. S. and Rogers, A. L.: Medical Mycology Manual. Burgess, Minneapolis, 1980, with permission.)

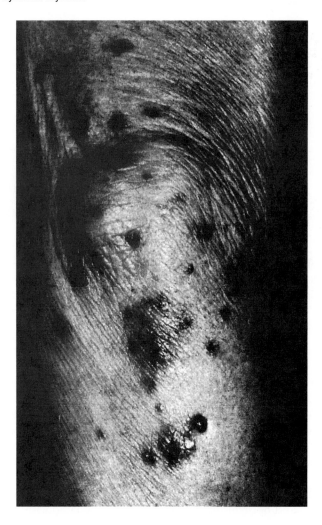

Figure 7–4. Pustular eruptions of knee, hematogenous spread from internal organs to skin (secondary cutaneous blastomycosis). (From Musial, C. E., et al: Recovery of *blastomyces dermatitidis* from blood of a patient with disseminated blastomycosis. J Clin Microbiol 1987, with permission.)

ganism is isolated from blood cultures (Musial et al. 1987), supporting the hematogenous route of dissemination. Interestingly, this fungus is uncommon in AIDS patients.

Without therapy consisting of amphotericin B or the azoles (see Module 2), the prognosis is poor.

COCCIDIOIDES IMMITIS (Fig. 7–5)

Culture: On SABHI agar at room temperature or 37°C, a moist white colony initially forms that is later covered with white fluffy mycelium (see Color Plate 71). Colonies form in 5 to 7 days, although diagnostic arthroconidia require about 2 weeks. *Coccidioides* colonies can be grown on bacteriology sheep blood agar or chocolate agar plates set up on a routine sputum for bacteria. Sniffing these plates could be dangerous, as the fungus is highly contagious.

Microscopic: Tease mounts of the colony reveal hyphal branching at 90-degree angles and many THICK-WALLED, BARREL-SHAPED or rectangular ARTHROCONIDIA ALTERNATING WITH EMPTY DISJUNCTOR CELLS. The opportunists *Gymnoascus uncinatus*, *Auxarthron* sp. and *Malbranchea* sp. also produce alternating arthroconidia, and *Geotrichum candidum* and *Trichosporon* sp. (see Module 5) produce adjacent arthroconidia. Demonstration of spherules with endospores being released is therefore required for final identification, or a positive immunodiffusion test using known antibodies to *Coccidioides immitis* and extract of the unknown mold as antigen (exoantigen test).

The tissue phase of this organism may be grown only under special in vitro conditions or animal inoculations. Round, THICK-WALLED SPHERULES (sporangia) filled with small ENDOSPORES are observed on conversion and also on specimen direct mounts (see Color Plate 67). Young spherules with undeveloped endospores may resem-

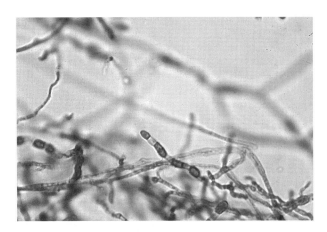

Figure 7–5. Mold phase, *Coccidioides immitis*, LPCB stain (magnification ×450).

ble yeast cells of *B. dermatitidis*. With a Vaseline-sealed coverslip over the specimen, spherules form multiple germ tubes after a 24-hour incubation at 37°C, while *Blastomyces* exhibits only broad-based single-budding cells.

Pathogenicity: C. immitis produces coccidioidomycosis.

COCCIDIOIDO-MYCOSIS (SAN JOAQUIN FEVER) (Fig. 7–6)

Coccidioidomycosis, caused by *C. immitis,* is endemic in the desert areas of the southwestern United States, with some cases reported from Central and South America. The arthroconidia are very resistant to heat, dryness, and salinity. They reside in the soil; 10 to 14 days after breathing contaminated dust, 60% of patients with coccidioidomycosis exhibit an asymptomatic respiratory infection. The remaining 40% present symptoms of mild or, rarely, severe flulike respiratory illness (primary pulmonary coccidioidomycosis). The patient recovers or, if the immune response is compromised, may succumb to gradual or rapid disseminated disease. In endemic areas, 3% of the normal population converts to a positive *Coccidioides* skin test every year. However, over 20% of AIDS patients develop clinically apparent coccidioidal infection every year (Galgiani et al. 1990). Pulmonary complications such as cavity formation or persistent pneumonia occur in 5% of adults, especially those with pre-existing lung disease or diabetes mellitus. Organisms may spread hematogenously from the lungs to the bones, joints, skin, subcutaneous tissues, internal organs, brain, and lymph nodes (Smith et al. 1994). The skin, musculoskeletal system, and central nervous system are the most common sites of invasion.

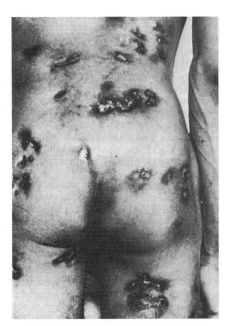

Figure 7–6. Disseminated coccidioidomycosis. (From Rippon, J. W.: Medical Mycology. WB Saunders, Philadelphia, 1988, with permission.)

Coccidioidal infections in AIDS patients are typically quite progressive compared to immunocompetent patients, as cell-mediated immunity is important in combating this fungus. There is also a question whether the asymptomatic infection from an earlier exposure reactivates with a decrease in helper T cells below 200 cells/mm^3. Diffuse pulmonary infiltrates and hematogenous dissemination are common (Galgiani et al. 1994). The prognosis is good for primary pulmonary disease, but disseminated mycosis can be fatal. Amphotericin B, the azoles, and a new azole SCH 39304 are variably effective (Hostetler et al. 1994); the patient's immune capability is more important.

HISTOPLASMA CAPSULATUM
(Figs. 7–7 and 7–8)

Culture: On brain heart infusion agar with blood at room temperature, the slow-growing colony is initially moist and later develops a low, white to brown aerial mycelium. The texture of mature colonies may be glabrous, velvety, or woolly (see Color Plate 72). Once the colony has initially formed on brain heart infusion agar with blood, transfer it to a less nutritious medium, for example, SABHI agar, so that characteristic microscopic structures will develop.

On brain heart infusion agar with blood at 37°C, a rough, mucoid, cream to tan colony forms (see Color Plate 73). Several transfers may be necessary to convert the mold to yeast phase.

Microscopic: Tease mounts of the room temperature MOLD phase from SABHI agar reveal conidiophores at 90-degree angles to the hyphae, which support large round MACROCONIDIA (chlamydoconidia) with smooth, spiny, or FINLIKE (tuberculate) EDGES. Small, round to teardrop, smooth or rough MICROCONIDIA are along the sides of the hyphae. Variants may be observed where macroconidia alone, microconidia alone, or sterile hyphae are present. *Histoplasma capsulatum* macroconidia closely resem-

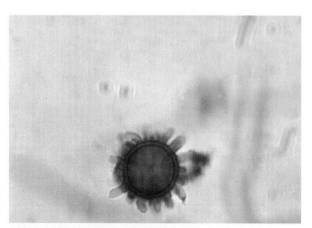

Figure 7–7. Macroconidium mold phase, *Histoplasma capsulatum*, LPCB stain (magnification ×1000).

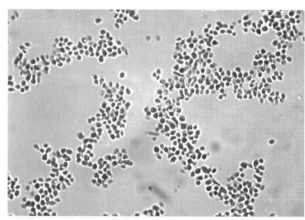

Figure 7–8. Yeast phase, *Histoplasma capsulatum*, LPCB stain (magnification ×450).

ble those of the opportunists *Sepedonium* sp. and rough-walled *Chrysosporium* sp. (see Module 3). However, *Histoplasma* is slow growing and can be converted to a yeast phase, while the opportunists are rapid growing and do not possess a yeast phase.

The 37°C yeast phase microscopically appears as SMALL, single-budding YEAST cells.

Pathogenicity: H. capsulatum causes histoplasmosis.

HISTOPLASMOSIS (DARLING'S DISEASE) (Fig. 7–9)

Histoplasmosis, caused by *Histoplasma capsulatum*, is endemic in the Mississippi River area, the Ohio River valley, and along the Appalachian Mountains, although it has been reported throughout the world. The organisms multiply in bird droppings, including chicken droppings and bat guano. Interestingly, the fungus lives in the gastrointestinal tract of bats. Birds do not get infected because of their high body temperature, which inhibits fungal tissue invasion (Rinaldi 1990). Wind seems to be the common vector for transporting infectious particles in actively disturbed, contaminated soil. The disease is not contagious or transmissible from human to human, or animal to human. Except for direct inoculation into the skin, all infections result from inhalation of the mold form of the fungus. Of all infections, 90 to 95% are asymptomatic or subclinical, with a self-limiting respiratory flulike illness. This common type of histoplasmosis has resulted in a positive skin test for most of the people in endemic areas. Occasionally the patient may experience an acute pulmonary form of disease, associated with night sweats, cough, fever, and weight loss. In a few instances, a chronic cavitary pulmonary disease occurs with productive cough and radiograph signs resembling cavitary tuberculosis. Also in a few patients, the pulmonary infection disseminates by way of the blood to the adrenals, spleen, liver, kidneys, skin, oral mucosa, eye, central nervous system, and other organs. Disseminated histoplasmosis manifests as a moderately chronic disease in immune competent individuals, but as a rapidly fulminant disease in immunocompromised patients.

As many as 53% of AIDS patients from endemic areas develop histoplasmosis. In addition, cases from nonendemic localities are now being reported (Rinaldi 1990). Predominant findings are fever (69%), weight loss (50%), splenomegaly (33%), and adenopathy (24%). Laboratory abnormalities include anemia (96%), leukopenia (61%), and thrombocytopenia (40%). On chest radiographs, interstitial infiltrates are seen in 51% of affected AIDS patients compared to 33% of normal hosts (Graybill 1990). Although infiltrates are a common finding on chest radiographs, respiratory symptoms are not predominant in AIDS cases. Recovery of organisms on culture is best if biopsy culture is obtained from the most affected organ. If there are no localizing signs, frequently the fungal burden is so dense that a simple Wright-Giemsa stain of a peripheral blood smear shows the characteristic pseudo-encapsulated yeast (tissue) form in monocytes. Blood cultures are frequently positive, especially if processed by lysis centrifugation (DuPont Isolator).

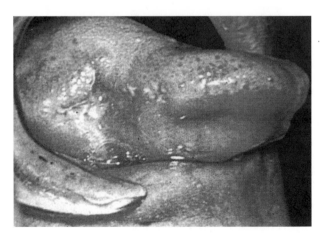

Figure 7–9. Histoplasmosis of tongue. (From Beneke, E. S.: Human Mycoses. Upjohn, Kalamazoo, 1984, with permission.)

Therapy with amphotericin B in a normal, immunocompetent host brings the mortality from disseminated histoplasmosis down to less than 10% as compared to 80% mortality in untreated hosts. However, in immunocompromised individuals, results are discouraging, and frequent relapses occur with the cessation of therapy. The azoles are less toxic, but relapses are still a significant problem.

PARACOCCIDIOIDES BRASILIENSIS (Figs. 7–10 and 7–11)

Culture: On SABHI agar at room temperature, colonies grow slowly—2 cm in 3 weeks. They are smooth at first and later become covered with white to tan aerial mycelium (see Color Plate 74).

On brain heart infusion agar with blood at 37°C, colonies are waxy, wrinkled, and cream to tan colored (see Color Plate 75). Conversion to the yeast phase requires 3 to 7 days.

Microscopic: Tease mounts of the room temperature mold colony show mostly hyphae with intercalary and terminal chlamydoconidia. Occasionally conidia resembling *B. dermatitidis* and *Chrysosporium* sp. are observed. Arthroconidia may form.

The 37°C YEAST phase microscopically appears as large, THICK-WALLED, MULTIPLE BUDDING yeast cells with narrow necks where the daughter cells attach. This form has the likeness of a SHIP'S WHEEL.

Pathogenicity: P. brasiliensis causes paracoccidioidomycosis.

PARACOCCIDIOIDO-MYCOSIS (SOUTH AMERICAN BLASTOMYCOSIS) (Fig. 7–12)

Paracoccidioidomycosis, caused by *P. brasiliensis,* is endemic in South America, especially Brazil. Organisms are saprobic, living in soil, in water, or on plants. The fungal mold form is typically inhaled, producing pulmonary lesions similar to tuberculosis and other mycoses (pulmonary paracoccidioidomycosis). Less commonly, the oral mucosa and gums become infected following trauma caused by chewing contaminated vegetable

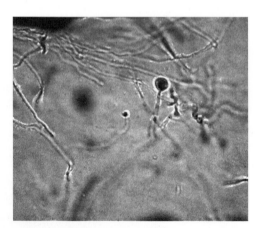

Figure 7–10. Conidium, mold phase, *Paracoccidioides brasilienesis,* LPCB stain (magnification ×450).

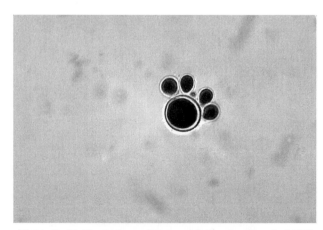

Figure 7–11. Yeast phase, *Paracoccidioides brasiliensis,* LPCB stain (magnification ×450).

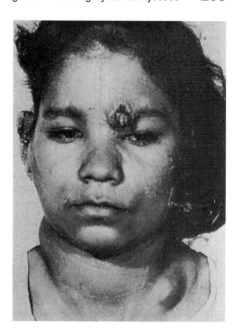

Figure 7–12. Cutaneous paracoccidioidomycosis with enlarged lymph nodes. (From Rippon, J. W.: Medical Mycology. WB Saunders, Philadelphia, 1988, with permission.)

matter. Crusted ulcers develop, which may spread to adjacent tonsils, nasal mucosa, and face (mucocutaneous paracoccidioidomycosis). Fungi from the oral ulcers or contaminated food are swallowed and cause intestinal manifestations, which may spread to adjacent structures such as liver, spleen, and adrenals (visceral paracoccidioidomycosis). Lymph node enlargement is quite notable in each of the disease manifestations, and lymph node biopsy represents a good source of specimens for cultures and stains. Patients expire in 2 or 3 years from disseminated disease or malnourishment from the inability to eat. Several cases of this fungal infection have been reported in AIDS patients, although primarily only in endemic countries. It is rare in AIDS patients from nonendemic locations (San-Blas 1993).

Therapy consists of trimethoprim plus sulfamethexazole or the new azoles. With acute disease, *P. brasiliensis* IgM is elevated, whereas in chronic disease, *P. brasiliensis* IgA is elevated. Both decrease with therapy, and the levels can be followed to determine cure (Blotta and Camargo 1993).

FINAL EXAM *Matching: Place the letter of the fungus from* Column B *in front of the corresponding description in* Column A.

Column A

1. _____ Multiple budding yeast
2. _____ Spherules
3. _____ Alternating arthroconidia
4. _____ Tuberculate macroconidia
5. _____ Pseudo-encapsulated yeasts inside monocytes
6. _____ Broad-based, thick-walled, single-budding yeasts

Column B

_____ A. *Blastomyces dermatitidis* mold phase

_____ B. *Paracoccidioides brasiliensis* tissue phase

_____ C. *Histoplasma capsulatum* mold phase

_____ D. *Coccidioides immitis* tissue phase

_____ E. *Blastomyces dermatitidis* tissue phase

_____ F. *Histoplasma capsulatum* tissue phase

_____ G. *Coccidioides immitis* mold phase

7. Discuss two safety precautions that should be met when working with the mold forms of systemic pathogens.

8. When changing a dimorphic mold to the yeast phase, what are two conditions necessary for complete conversion?

9. Compare and contrast:

   A. *Blastomyces dermatitidis*, *Chrysosporium* sp., and *Scedosporium apiospermum*

   B. *Coccidioides immitis* and *Geotrichum candidum*

Matching. Place the letter of the answer from Column B in front of the disease in Column A. An answer may be used more than once, as may the disease.

Column A	Column B
10. _____ Coccidioidomycosis	_____ A. Mainly in S. America
11. _____ Histoplasmosis	_____ B. Conidia in desert soil
12. _____ Paracoccidioidomycosis	_____ C. Associated with San Joaquin Valley, California
13. _____ Blastomycosis	_____ D. Fungi found in bird droppings phase
	_____ E. Mainly in Mississippi and Ohio River valleys

For the next three questions, refer to this case study.

A 40-year-old woman from Washington, D.C., was admitted to the hospital for investigation of a mass in her right lung. She was on chemotherapy and the cancer seemed to be going into remission. There were no complaints outside those associated with anti-cancer medication, except that she possessed a slight chronic cough. Past history revealed a flulike illness 6 weeks prior to admission, while she was visiting her sister in California. X-rays showed a well-delineated round density in the right lower lobe. A skin test for tuberculosis was negative. The nodule was surgically removed, and some of the specimen was sent for mycology culture. Within 4 days, a white fluffy mold grew well on both plain SABHI agar and media with cycloheximide and chloramphenicol.

14. What disease do you suspect? Circle the correct letter.

A. Fungus ball with *Scedosporium apiospermum*

B. Abscess with *Candida albicans*

C. Pulmonary coccidioidomycosis

D. *Trichophyton mentagrophytes* infection

E. Infection due to *Geotrichum candidum*

F. Histoplasmosis

15. What criteria in the patient's clinical picture and past history would support this diagnosis? List two.

16. Which two procedures must you perform to confirm the diagnosis, and what would be the results?

For the next four questions, refer to this case study.

A 5-year-old girl from a farm town in Ohio was admitted to the regional hospital for suspected tuberculosis. She possessed a chronic cough with productive sputum, and she complained of breathlessness, tiredness, and weight loss over the last several months. Multiple sputum specimens showed no acid-fast bacilli; her tuberculin skin test was negative. Abnormal hematologic findings were anemia, a low white blood cell count, and some monocytes containing intracellular yeasts with a narrow isthmus between mother and daughter cells. Blood specimens were drawn into a Dupont Isolator, processed, and placed on brain heart infusion agar with blood at room temperature. After 3 weeks, tan, fluffy colonies formed. Microscopically, the fungus produced only microconidia along the sides of the hyphae.

17. What disease do you suspect and why? Give two reasons.

18. How would you confirm the identity of this isolate? Present two ways.

19. What was the probable mode of exposure to the etiologic agent?

20. An opportunistic fungus is morphologically similar to the characteristic structures of the causative organism. Name it and provide two ways it may be differentiated from the disease agent in this case study.

STOP HERE UNTIL YOU HAVE COMPLETED THE QUESTIONS.

Look up the answers in the back of the book. If you missed more than three, go back and review this module.

Answers for Study Questions and Final Exams

MODULE 1

II. A. 4. Study questions, page 9.
1. F   Plants contain chlorophyll; fungi do not.
2. Yeasts. The sputum came from body temperature (37°C). At 37°C, a dimorphic organism is in a yeast phase.
3. Nodular organs
4. D

II. B. 1. c. Study questions, pages 17–18.
1. A
2. T
3. F   *Candida albicans* forms chlamydospores, which are nongerminating vesicles.
4. D
5. E
6. A. Sporangiospore
   B. Columella
   C. Sporangiophore

VI. Final exam, pages 24–26.
1. A. Zygosporangium (or zygospore inside zygosporangium)
   B. Blastoconidia
   C. Racquet hyphae
   D. Macroconidium
   E. Verrucose topography
   F. Ascospore
   G. Vegetative hyphae
   H. Sessile chlamydoconidium
   I. Granular or powdery texture
   J. Dimorphism
   K. Basidiospore
   L. Arthroconidia

2. Velvety to woolly texture; umbonate and rugose topography; front color white with a white peripheral ring; reverse colors (starting from the periphery and moving inward) white, orange, yellow-orange, orange-tan, yellow-orange, center orange-tan OR white peripheral rings, with inner rings of varying shades of orange (yellow-orange, orange, and orange-tan). A reasonable facsimile of the above will suffice for an answer.
3. C
4. Phialoconidia, anamorph, deuteromycota
5. D
   G
   C

MODULE 2

II. C. Study questions, pages 36–37.
1. Any three of these answers are acceptable:
   • Make sure the specimen is collected from the area most likely to be affected.
   • Use sterile technique in collecting the specimen.
   • The specimen must be adequate.
   • The specimen must be delivered promptly to the laboratory.
   • The laboratory must process the specimen quickly.
   • The specimen must be adequately labelled.

2. T
3. Overnight incubation and multiplication of fungi in the bladder will increase the chance of isolating them on culture.
4. D
5. F Alcohol removes surface contaminants; it does not affect fungal pathogens.
6. F Many times even with concentration, the fungus won't grow.
7. T
8. F Granules are composed of organisms (bacteria, funguslike bacteria, or fungi) with or without a cementlike matrix or a center of necrotic material. They are the most likely source for isolating the etiologic agent of the infection.

III. I. Study questions, page 49.

1. Any two of the following answers are adequate:
   - A direct exam allows you to send out an immediate preliminary report to the physician, so he or she may initiate treatment or look for other diagnoses.
   - With the direct exam results, you will know whether to inoculate any special media.
   - The direct exam allows you to observe the yeast phase of dimorphic organisms.
   - The direct exam may provide a clue as to the identity of the causative agent, without having to wait for the fungus to incubate.
2. D
3. A
4. F
5. B
6. G
7. E
8. F All bacteria and fungi will stand out against the black background. Look only for encapsulated organisms.
9. D
10. F The phenol in LPCB kills any fungus that may be present; thus, it cannot be cultured.

IV. E. Study questions, page 57.

1. B DTM and cycloheximide inhibit fungal opportunists. BHIB will be overgrown by bacteria, making isolation of opportunists difficult.

2. D While all these media may grow *Histoplasma,* fastidious strains require media with blood as extra nutrition. Additionally, because sputum has many bacteria and fungal opportunists that would overrun the slower growing *Histoplasma,* the medium should contain inhibitory antibiotics.
3. A While SABHI will also grow yeasts, bacteria will overrun the culture; therefore use gentamicin and chloramphenicol. Do not use cycloheximide as it will inhibit yeasts.
4. D SABHI, IMA, and birdseed agar will all grow *C. neoformans.* However, bacteria and other yeasts may obscure its growth. Birdseed agar will show dark brown colonies that stand out.
5. Intermediate growth means that a mature colony forms in 6–10 days.
6. T

VII. Final exam, pages 66–67.

1. A 24-hour collection becomes easily overgrown with bacterial contaminants and fungal opportunists.
2. Any two of the following:
   Coccidioides immitis
   Histoplasma capsulatum
   Actinomyces
   Nocardia
   Candida
   Cryptococcus neoformans
   Opportunists repeatedly isolated
3. F Unlike bacteria, fungi do not make the broth cloudy. This necessitates frequent Gram staining.
4. Chitin
5. There are three possible answers for this question, depending on the individual's philosophy and the laboratory's economic situation.

    Some laboratories incubate all their cultures at room temperature, so a costly incubator is not required. Fungi will grow at this temperature, but it takes longer for them to mature and thus identify.

    If all cultures are put at 30°C, they will grow faster, thus aiding quick results, but an incubator is necessary. A 30°C temperature is recommended in this module.

Some laboratories incubate one set of cultures at 37°C to isolate the yeast phase of dimorphic fungi, and a second set of cultures at room temperature or 30°C for other organisms. This is probably not cost effective since so few dimorphic fungi are isolated. Also the yeast phase could be immediately observed in specimen direct mounts.

6.   *Advantages*

Tease mount—Quick to make; no incubation period

Slide culture—Beautiful conidial juxtaposition; 2 mounts from one slide culture

Coverslip sandwich—Beautiful conidial juxtaposition; several mounts from one plate

         Disadvantages

Tease mount—May destroy conidial juxtaposition

Slide culture—Takes time to set up; incubation period required

Coverslip sandwich—Incubation period required

7. **Specimen site**—Since you know that only certain organisms can be isolated from a particular specimen (see Chart 2–2), many fungi are ruled out.

Colonial morphology—Sometimes a colony has such a characteristic morphology, for example, *Penicillium*, that you suspect its identity even before observing the microscopic characteristics.

General microscopic morphology— Since you know that only certain organisms possess hyphae, yeast forms, filamentous bacterial characteristics, or dimorphic attributes (see Chart 2–4), many fungi are ruled out.

VIII. F. Study questions—Supplemental Rationale, pages 71–72.

1. B
2. A—both
   B—both
   C—antigen
   D—both
3. Causes of false (+): Any three of the following:
 • *Trichosporon* infection
 • collagen vascular disease
 • malignancy
 • rheumatoid arthritis

• syneresis fluid
• complement

Ways to decrease them: Any one of the following:
 • heat inactivation of nonspecific interference and complement
 • pronase pretreatment
 • 2-β-mercaptoethanol pretreatment
 • removal of syneresis fluid from agar plates before taking colonies for testing

4. A known luminescent labelled single-stranded DNA probe to the organism in question is allowed to hybridize with ribosomal RNA from a sonicated fungal culture. If the fungus in question is present, the fungal rRNA will combine with the probe DNA and luminesce.

5. Distilled water, freezing, lyophilization, oil overlay

6. Polyene macrolides—amp B (systemic), nystatin (yeast)

 Pyrimidine analogues—5FC (yeast)

 Azoles—clotrimazole, miconazole ketoconazole, itraconazole, fluconazole (systemic, yeast, dermatophytes)

 Griseofulvin (dermatophytes)

 Allylamines—naftifine, terbinafine (dermatophytes)

7. Because the immune system isn't there to help fight infection, and also patients are frequently granulocytopenic, antifungal agents alone only temporarily work, with frequent relapses and eventually antifungal drug resistance.

MODULE 3

III. D. Study questions, page 87.

1. Any five of these answers will suffice:
 • Most fungal opportunists form mature colonies in four to five days.
 • They live in the soil.
 • They become airborne occasionally.
 • They are normally inhaled.
 • Respiratory specimens may normally yield a few colonies of fungal opportunists.
 • Fungal opportunists may be normal skin flora.
 • They may contaminate laboratory cultures.

- Opportunists are usually nonpathogenic.
- They are opportunistic pathogens in debilitated patients.
- Antibiotics in fungal media inhibit fungal opportunists.
- Fungal opportunists must be repeatedly isolated in large numbers from cultured patient specimens to be considered the causative agent of a disease.

2. A. Sporangium
   B. Rhizoid
   C. Stolon

IV. A. 9. Study questions, page 96.

1. *Stemphylium* sp.
2. B,D,F,G
3. C Black yeast
   E Shield cells
   F Enlarged central cell
   C Arthroconidia
   A Single, one-celled, black conidia

IV. B. 10. Study questions, page 105.

1. Any three of the following will suffice:
   - *Gliocladium* forms balls of conidia; the rest produce chains.
   - *Paecilomyces* exhibits tapering conidiophores; the rest do not.
   - *Scopulariopsis* conidia are lemon shaped; the rest are round.
   - *Scopulariopsis* colonies are tan; the rest are usually shades of green.
   - All except *Gliocladium* have been numerously reported as human pathogens.

2. B   Aseptate
   A,B Vesicles
   C   Blastoconidia
   B   Merosporangia
   A   Foot cells
   A   Phialides

3. F *Acremonium* exhibits unbranching, gradually tapering conidiophores with balls of conidia.

4. B   *Chrysosporium*
   B,C *Sepedonium*
   D,E *Scedosporium apiospermum*
   A   *Blastomyces dermatitidis*
   A,C *Histoplasma capsulatum*

V. Final exam, pages 110–113.

1. D
2. F Dematiaceous organisms exhibit dark-colored hyphae and/or conidia.
3. A,C 1.
   A,B 2.
   A   3.

4. Any two of the following:
   - *Epicoccum* has sporodchia, while *Ulocladium* possesses a bent-knee conidiophore, and *Stemphylium* has a straight conidiophore.
   - *Epicoccum* produces orange colonies; the others produce black ones.
   - *Stemphylium* conidial cross septa are constricted; those in the other two fungi are not.

5. F *Bipolaris* possesses the bent-knee conidiophore, while that of *Helminthosporium* is straight. Since the poroconidia are so similar, *Bipolaris* was often misidentified as *Helminthosporium* in the past.

6. T
7. A. *Curvularia* sp.
   B. *Syncephalastrum* sp.
   C. *Penicillium* sp.
   D. *Mucor* sp.
   E. *Scopulariopsis* sp.
   F. *Acremonium* sp.
   G. *Aspergillus* sp.
   H. *Cladosporium* sp.
   I. *Alternaria* sp.
   J. *Paecilomyces* sp.
   K. *Rhizopus* sp.
   L. *Aureobasidium* sp.

8. T
9. A
10. F The cornea is usually resistant to infection; keratomycosis primarily begins with trauma to the eye.
11. Zygomycosis. Uncontrolled diabetes is the typical predisposing factor. Infection characteristically begins in the nasal passages or eye, and aseptate hyphae indicate the fungus must be of the phylum Zygomycota.
12. C
13. *Rhizopus* sp.
14. Absolutely not. This disease rapidly erodes into surrounding blood vessels, with systemic spread and death within 10 days after the initial sinus/eye symptoms. Treatment should begin as soon as the disease is suspected.

MODULE 4

II. E. Study questions, page 122.

1. E
2. A,D
3. B,F
4. C

III. A. 6 Study questions, page 127.
1. D   endothrix invasion
2. Athlete's foot
3. *Microsporum*
4. F   Dermatophytes are intermediate to slow growers.
5. T
6. B,C,E

III. B. 3. b. Study questions, page 136.
1. A,C,E
2. B
3. C
4. F   *E. floccosum* macroconidia are club shaped; *T. verrucosum* are rat-tail.

V. Final exam, pages 139–141.
1. Superficial mycoses elicit little pathology, while cutaneous mycoses involve more tissue destruction.
2. T
3. B
4. E
5. Any two of the following will suffice:
   - *T. verrucosum* grows poorly at 25°C; *T. violaceum* grows well.
   - *T. verrucosum* colonies are white to bright yellow; *T. violaceum* colonies are violet.
   - On thiamine-enriched media, *T. verrucosum* forms rare rat-tailed macroconidia, while *T. violaceum* does not form macroconidia.
   - Many strains of *T. verrucosum* require inositol as well as thiamine; *T. violaceum* requires only thiamine.
   - *T. verrucosum* produces an ectothrix hair invasion, while *T. violaceum* produces an endothrix invasion.
6. B
7. C,D,E,F
8. C
9. D
10. B
11. B
12. D
13. E

MODULE 5

II. B. 4. Study questions, pages 153–154.
1. C
2. D
3. C
4. F
5. B
6. A
7. *Candida albicans*

II. B. 7. Study questions, page 157.
1. F   Most, but not all, isolates of *C. albicans* form germ tubes and chlamydospores.
2. F   A pseudohypha is constricted; a germ tube is not.
3. D,F,G
4. A,C,D
5. A,D,E
6. A,D
7. *Rhodotorula*
8. *Geotrichum candidum*

IV. Final exam, pages 162–163.
1. D
2. Any three of the answers below:
   - Pigeon breeder. *Cryptococcus* is frequently found in pigeon droppings.
   - Patient was immunosuppressed, so his host defenses were lower than normal.
   - Central nervous system symptoms. *Cryptococcus* has a predilection for the brain and meninges.
   - Mucoid yeast. Mucoid colonies are composed of encapsulated organisms.
   - Inhibited by cycloheximide and chloramphenicol.

   How are the other answers ruled out?
   - *Candida.* Organisms would be seen on Gram stain.
   - No disease. *Anything* from CSF should be investigated, whether you think it is a laboratory contaminant or not. In this case, once the yeast is identified, there would be no question as to its significance.
   - *Histoplasma.* Possibly, since it is associated with bird droppings and is endemic in the Midwest. However, in CSF, you would see small pseudoencapsulated yeasts *inside* phagocytic cells. Also, at 30°C, *Histoplasma* is a slow-growing mold.
   - *Coccidioides.* This has a predilection for the brain, but in CSF you would observe spherules, and at 30°C a white mold rapidly grows.
3. The capsule around *Cryptococcus* inhibits stain uptake by the yeast itself (Gram stain, see Module 2), thus making it barely visible. When seen, it also resembles debris.
4. Any three of the following: caffeic

acid agar, assimilations, urease, India ink preparation, mucicarmine stain.

5. B
6. D

MODULE 6

II. C. Study questions, pages 180–182.

1. B   *C. carrionii* produces black dots or sclerotic bodies; *C. trichoides* causes phaeohyphomycosis, in which no black dots are observed.

2. Similarities. Any three of the following:
   - Black yeasts at first
   - Annellides, although they are not uniformly accepted for *Wangiella*
   - Terminal balls of conidia, which tend to fall down the sides of the conidiophore
   - Clusters of conidia may form on short denticles off the sides of the hyphae.
   - Both may cause phaeohypho-mycosis.

   Differences. Any three of the following:
   - *E. jeanselmei* uses nitrate, while *Wangiella* does not.
   - *Wangiella* grows at 42°C; *E. jeanselmei* can not.
   - *E. jeanselmei* may cause mycetoma and keratomycosis, while *Wangiella* has not been a reported agent of these infections.
   - *Wangiella* does not exhibit annellides as the most distinct, stable, and unique form.

3. B,D,F
4. A
5. C
6. Cleistothecia with asci and ascospores
7. T

IV. Final exam, pages 189–191.

1. C,D (also conidia of B)
2. A
3. B,C
4. B,C
5. A
6. F   Bacteria also may form them.
7. C   The answer cannot be D, because in actinomycosis, granules are yellow.
8. Two of the following:
   - *Sporothrix* colonies turn black with age, especially on potato dextrose agar; *Acremonium* colonies do not.
   - *Sporothrix* possesses a yeast phase; *Acremonium* does not.
   - The mold phase of *Sporothrix* is not as tightly packed in the flowerette as *Acremonium*
   - *Sporothrix* does not cause mycetoma; *Acremonium* may.

9. E   Although *Fonsecaea pedrosoi* and *Fonsecaea compacta* commonly exhibit polymorphism, *C. carrionii* may produce phialides with phialoconidia on certain media.

10. 1. B   Casein, tyrosine, xanthine
    2. C   Gelatin liquefaction
    3. D   KOH prep for sclerotic bodies
    4. A   Catalase, fermentations

11. T
12. T
13. T

14. Any two of the following:
    - Mycetoma invades bone; chromoblastomycosis does not.
    - Chromoblastomycosis exhibits dry lesions; mycetoma demonstrates draining sinuses.
    - Black sclerotic bodies are seen in chromoblastomycosis, while in mycetoma, there are variously colored granules. Black granules of mycetoma differ from black sclerotic bodies in that the granules are composed of chlamydoconidia with occasional hyphae.
    - Different etiologic agents, plus mycetoma, may be eumycotic or actinomycotic.

15. B   *Actinomyces* is normal flora of the oral cavity, while the other diseases are produced by exogenous organisms introduced by skin puncture with contaminated thorns and so forth.

16. Sporotrichosis. Any two of these reasons:
    - Lesions following the lymphatics
    - Cigar bodies in stained sections
    - Cream-colored colony at room temperature, which turned black with age
    - Black necrotic lesions

17. C   E is *Acremonium,* which appears similar but does not possess a yeast phase. A is wrong because this would be observed only at 37°C.

18. Since he is a rose gardener, the

patient probably was pricked with a contaminated thorn.

19. Chromoblastomycosis. Any two of the following:
    - Sclerotic bodies
    - Cauliflower lesions
    - A slow-growing organism with only this conidial arrangement is seen exclusively in chromoblasto-mycosis.

20. E   It cannot be A because *C. trichoides* causes phaeohyphomycosis, in which there are no sclerotic bodies or cauliflower lesions.

MODULE 7

III. Final exam, pages 203–205.

1. B
2. D
3. G
4. C
5. F
6. E
7. Any two of the following is acceptable:
    - Use slanted media in capped tubes rather than plated media. This minimizes the risk of conidia becoming airborne.
    - Wear mask and gloves.
    - Always work under a microbiologic hood.
    - Formalinize or wet down mold cultures before preparing tease mounts.
    - Never make slide cultures with the mold forms of systemic fungi; the conidia are too easily distributed into the air.
8. Any two of the following will suffice:
    - The medium must be enriched.
    - The medium must be kept moist.
    - The temperature should be 37°C.
    - The organisms must be subcultured onto fresh media several times for complete conversion.
9. A   All three fungi possess conidia on the sides or tips of the hyphae, resembling lollipops, and they all have white colonies. Here are some differences:
    - *Blastomyces* is a slow grower, while *Chrysosporium* is a rapid grower and *Scedosporium* is an intermediate grower.
    - *Blastomyces* has a yeast phase, while the others do not.
    - *Chrysosporium* is a nonpathogenic opportunist, while *Blastomyces* may cause systemic disease, and *Scedosporium* may produce subcutaneous problems.
    - *Scedosporium* has a rather commonly observed sexual stage. *Blastomyces* possesses a sexual stage, but it is not as routinely observed. *Chrysosporium* does not exhibit one.
    - *Scedosporium* and *Chrysosporium* are inhibited by cycloheximide and chloramphenicol (C&C); *Blastomyces* mold forms are not.

    B   Both organisms produce arthroconidia, are rapid growers, form white colonies, and may produce systemic disease. However, *Coccidioides* forms alternating arthroconidia, is not inhibited by C&C, and has a tissue phase, while *Geotrichum* forms adjacent arthroconidia, is inhibited by C&C, and possesses no tissue phase.
10. B,C
11. D,E
12. A
13. E
14. C   All five organisms grow relatively rapidly and are white; however, *Scedosporium* and *Geotrichum* are inhibited by cycloheximide, *Candida* is a yeast, and *Trichophyton* would cause dermatophytosis rather than a respiratory infection.
15. Any two of the following:
    - Patient on chemotherapy and therefore immunosuppressed
    - Flu was probably a mild case of coccidioidomycosis.
    - California: *Coccidioides* loves the desert soil there.
16. Any two of the following:
    - Perform LPCB tease mounts of the mold, under a microbiologic hood, and search for barrel-shaped arthroconidia alternating with empty cells.
    - Demonstrate spherules with endospores in histologic sections from the surgical specimen.
    - DNA probe or serologic studies with known antibodies, to identify the mold.

- Acute and convalescent sera to test for a fourfold rise in antibody titer to *Coccidioides.*

17. *Histoplasma capsulatum.* Any two of the following:
    - Ohio, endemic for histoplasmosis
    - Symptoms (chronic cough, breathlessness, tiredness, weight loss)
    - Typical yeasts on blood differential; they should rule out yeasts of *Blastomyces*
    - Slow grower on nutritious medium

18. Any two of the following:
    - Subculture the isolate to less nutritious medium like SABHI agar to see if the mold produces characteristic macroconidia.
    - Convert the fungus from the mold to yeast phase.
    - DNA probe or serologic studies with known antibodies, to identify the mold

- Acute and convalescent sera to test for a fourfold rise in antibody titer to *Histoplasma*

19. Farm town—probably a lot of chickens. *Histoplasma* resides in bird droppings.

20. *Histoplasma* and *Sepedonium* both possess microconidia and macroconidia (some people argue that the microconidia of *Sepedonium* are just immature macronidia). However, *Histoplasma* is a slow grower and produces a yeast phase, mold forms are not inhibited by cycloheximide and chloramphenicol, and the fungus may elicit systemic disease; *Sepedonium* is a rapid grower, has no yeast phase, is inhibited by cycloheximide and chloramphenicol, and is usually a nonpathogenic opportunist.

APPENDIX

B

Common Synonyms

Synonym	*Currently Accepted Name*
Acrotheca sporulation	*Rhinocladiella*-like conidial formation
Allescheria boydii	*Pseudallescheria boydii*
Bifidobacterium eriksonii, B. adolescentis	*Bifidobacterium dentium*
Blastomyces brasiliensis	*Paracoccidioides brasiliensis*
Cephalosporium	*Acremonium*
Cerebral chromomycosis	Phaeohyphomycosis
Chromomycosis	Chromoblastomycosis
Cladosporiosis	Phaeohyphomycosis
Cladosporium bantianum	*Cladosporium trichoides*
Cladosporium werneckii	*Exophiala werneckii*
Exophiala dermatitidis	*Wangiella dermatitidis*
Helminthosporium	misidentified isolates of *Drechslera* or *Bipolaris*
Hormodendrum	*Cladosporium*
Madura foot	Mycetoma
Maduromycosis	Mycetoma
Monilia	*Candida*
Moniliasis	Candidosis, Candidiasis (both accepted names)
Monosporium apiospermum	*Scedosporium apiospermum*
Mucormycosis	Zygomycosis
Mycotic keratitis	Keratomycosis
Nocardia caviae	*Nocardia otitidiscaviarum*
Nocardia madurae	*Actinomadura madurae*
Nocardia pelletierii	*Actinomadura pelletierii*
North American blastomycosis	Blastomycosis
Penicilliosis	Hyalohyphomycosis
Petriellidium boydii	*Pseudallescheria boydii*
Phaeoannellomyces werneckii	*Exophiala werneckii*
Phaeomycotic cyst	Phaeohyphomycosis
Phialophora dermatitidis	*Wangiella dermatitidis*
Phialophora gougerotii	*Exophiala jeanselmei*
Phialophora jeanselmei	*Exophiala jeanselmei*
Phycomycosis	Zygomycosis
Pityrosporum orbiculare	*Malassezia furfur*
Pityrosporum ovale	*Malassezia furfur*
Ringworm	Dermatophytosis

Synonym	*Currently Accepted Name*
San Joaquin Valley fever	Coccidioidomycosis
Scedosporium inflatum	*Scedosporium prolificans*
South American blastomycosis	Paracoccidioidomycosis
Sterigmata (on *Aspergillus, Penicillium*)	Phialides
Tinea versicolor	Pityriasis versicolor
Tinea barbae, capitis, corporis, cruris, manuum, pedis & unguium	Dermatophytosis
Trichosporon capitatum, Geotrichum capitatum	*Blastoschizomyces capitatum*
Trichosporon cutaneum	*Trichosporon beigelii*
Xylohypha bantiana	*Cladosporium trichoides*

(Adapted from Odds, FC, et al: Nomenclature of fungal diseases: a report and recommendations from a subcommittee of the International Society for Human and Animal Mycology (ISHAM). J Med Vet Mycol 30:1, 1992.)

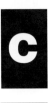
Glossary

TERM	DEFINITION
ACTINOMYCETE	All genera of the Actinomycetales except the family Mycobacteriaceae. Representative actinomycetes are *Nocardia, Streptomyces,* and *Actinomyces.*
ACTINOMYCOSIS	Disease caused by the anaerobic funguslike bacteria *Actinomyces, Bifidobacterium,* and *Arachnia.* The most common manifestations are facial (lumpy jaw), pulmonary, and abdominal. Draining sinus tracts contain characteristic sulfur-colored granules.
ACTINOMYCOTIC MYCETOMA	Mycetoma caused by a funguslike bacterium. Granules of various colors may be observed, depending on the etiologic agent.
AERIAL	Above the surface. Aerial hyphae usually support reproductive structures.
ANAMORPH	Asexual name.
ANNELLIDE	Tube- or vase-shaped conidiogenous cell. The first annelloconidium arises holoblastically, while the rest develop enteroblastically, from a tip which exhibits a new ring of material as each annelloconidium passes through. The outer rings provide a saw-toothed appearance at the annellide tip.
ANNELLOCONIDIUM	Conidium arising from an annellide. The first is holoblastic, but the rest develop enteroblastically. See drawing at ANNELLIDE.
ANNELLOPHORE	Conidiophore, or stalk, which supports annellides.
ANNULAR FRILL	Skirtlike remnant of parent material at the base of a conidium.
ANTHERIDIUM	Male sexual cell produced by the Ascomycota.

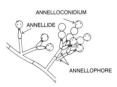

ANTIBODY	Protein synthesized by lymphocytes to help eliminate a foreign material (antigen) from the body.
ANTIGEN	Foreign material, including an organism or its extract, which will produce an immunologic response when inoculated into a suitable host.
APOPHYSIS	Swollen funnel-shaped columella.
ARTHRIC CONIDIOGENESIS	Thallic development whereby the daughter cells fragment within the hyphal strand before dispersing. They may be holoarthric or enteroarthric. See THALLIC CONIDIOGENESIS.
ARTHROCONIDIUM (pl. arthroconidia)	Arthric conidium produced by fragmentation of the hyphal strand through the septation points. Arthroconidia may form adjacent to each other or may be separated by disjunctor cells.
ARTHROSPORE	See ARTHROCONIDIUM.
ASCOCARP	Protective sac which houses asci and ascospores of molds in the Ascomycota. Asci are extruded from the ascocarp walls into the center of the sac. When the sac is ruptured, asci are released. If the intact sac is completely enclosed, it is called a cleistothecium.
ASCOGONIUM	Female sexual cell produced by members of the phylum Ascomycota.
ASCOMYCOTA	Fungal taxonomic phylum in which asci and ascospores are the sexual method of reproduction.
ASCOSPORE	Sexual spore formed by transfer of a male nucleus into a female cell and fusion of the nuclei into a zygote. The mother cell, or ascus, divides by meiosis so that 2, 4, or 8 ascospores develop inside. The asci may be surrounded by a protective outer ascocarp. See drawing at ASCOCARP.
ASCUS (pl. asci)	Sexual mother cell that forms ascospores inside and may be protected on the outside by an ascocarp. Asci are demonstrated in the phylum Ascomycota. See drawing at ASCOCARP.
ASEPTATE HYPHAE	Hyphae without cross-walls, so that nuclei and cytoplasm move freely between cells. Aseptate hyphae are found in the phylum Zygomycota.
ASEXUAL REPRODUCTION	Nuclear and cytoplasmic division, or mitosis, to produce two or more identical cells.
ASPERGILLOMA	Fungus ball caused by *Aspergillus*, especially *A. fumigatus* and *A. niger*.
ASPERGILLOSIS	A collection of opportunistic infections caused by various species of *Aspergillus*. The most important disease is invasive pulmonary aspergillosis, which initially demonstrates a lung focus, but later erodes into surrounding blood vessels and disseminates to the rest of the body.

IMMATURE MATURE

CLEISTOTHECIUM
ASCUS
ASCOSPORE

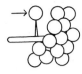

ASSIMILATION	Ability of a fungus to utilize a nutrient in the presence of oxygen.
BALLISTOCONIDIUM	Forcibly ejected conidium, usually triggered by a water droplet mechanism. Ballistoconidia, seen in the yeast *Sporobolomyces* sp., develop into individual colonies which satellite around the parent. To test for these projectiles, invert the plate of yeast colonies over a plate of fresh medium. Ballistoconidia will be discharged onto the new medium and form colonies after incubation.
BASIDIOCARP	Protective structure which houses basidia and basidiospores. The mushroom cap is a basidiocarp.
BASIDIOMYCOTA	Taxonomic phylum of fungi which produce basidiospores sexually.

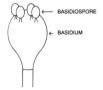

BASIDIOSPORE	Sexual spore formed by fusion of two compatible nuclei and cells into a zygote. Inside the mother cell, or basidium, the fused nuclei divide by meiosis to form four haploid nuclei, which later travel into four protrusions at the basidium tip to produce basidiospores. The basidium and basidiospores may be protected by an outer basidiocarp. These structures are observed in the phylum Basidiomycota.
BASIDIUM (pl. basidia)	Club-shaped mother cell from which basidiospores arise. Both structures are seen only in the phylum Basidiomycota. See drawing at BASIDIOSPORE.

BLACK DOT	Black sclerotic body found in chromoblastomycosis. This is to be differentiated from the black dot type of tinea capitis, produced by broken off infected hair shafts at the scalp surface.
BLACK PIEDRA	Stony black nodules around scalp hairs. The nodules are caused by *Piedraia hortai*.
BLASTIC CONIDIOGENESIS	Conidium formation whereby the parent cell enlarges, then a septum divides the enlarged portion into a daughter cell. The daughter begins to develop *before* it is separated from the parent. Blastic conidiogenesis may be holoblastic or enteroblastic.
BLASTOCONIDIUM (pl. blastoconidia)	Holoblastic conidium produced by budding. Yeasts are typical examples of blastoconidia, although some molds (for example, *Cladosporium, Aureobasidium,* and *Nigrospora*) also demonstrate them.
BLASTOMYCOSIS	Infection with *Blastomyces dermatitidis*. It initially manifests itself as a pulmonary disease, but if the patient is debilitated, infection may disseminate throughout the body, particularly bone and skin.
BLASTOSPORE	See BLASTOCONIDIUM.
CANDIDIASIS, CANDIDOSIS	Spectrum of diseases produced by the genus *Candida*. Usually infection is opportunistic; an upset in the balance of normal flora by antibiotics, anticancer drugs, debilitating illness, and so forth, enables *Candida* to proliferate where it once was held in check.

**CHLAMYDOCONIDIUM
(pl. chlamydoconidia)**

Thick-walled hyphal survival conidium during poor environmental conditions, which will germinate and produce conidia when a better climate occurs. In the past, chlamydospore was the general term; however, a chlamydospore neither germinates nor develops conidia when mature. Chlamydospores are observed in yeasts, while chlamydoconidia are seen in molds.

CHLAMYDOSPORE

Thick-walled vesicle of *Candida albicans* and some other yeasts, which neither germinates nor produces conidia when mature. See CHLAMYDOCONIDIUM.

CHROMOBLASTOMYCOSIS

Slow-progressing fungal infection of subcutaneous tissues, usually the extremities, with development of dark sclerotic bodies (black dots) on the tissue surfaces.

CIGAR BODY

Yeast form of *Sporothrix schenckii,* so called because it resembles the shape of a cigar.

CLAMP CONNECTION

Bridge between two adjacent hyphal cells whereby duplication of compatible nuclei takes place. Clamp connections are seen in the Basidiomycota as a part of the reproductive process.

**CLEISTOTHECIUM
(pl. cleistothecia)**

Completely enclosed ascocarp, containing asci and ascospores.

COCCIDIOIDOMYCOSIS

Infection with *Coccidioides immitis.* Initially, the disease presents as a flulike respiratory illness, but if the patient is debilitated, it may spread to the rest of the body, particularly the brain.

COLLARETTE

Small ring of remnant material, either at the tip of a phialide or base of a columella.

COLUMELLA (pl. collumellae)

Supporting structure at the tip of a sporangiophore and base of a sporangium. Most, but not all, zygomycetous fungi produce columellae.

CONDIDIOGENESIS

Conidium formation.

CONIDIOGENOUS CELL

Parent cell from which conidia directly arise. Annellides and phialides are examples of conidiogenous cells.

CONIDIOPHORE

Stalk on which conidia develop. A conidiophore may be a conidiogenous cell or may support conidiogenous cells.

CONIDIUM (pl. conidia)

Nonmotile, asexual reproductive structure which usually separates from the parent. It is not produced by cleavage, conjugation, or free-cell formation. See drawing at CONIDIOPHORE.

COTTONY TEXTURE

Colony with hyphae rising in the air, often an inch, before conidia develop. Opportunistic fungi may elicit cottony colonies; pathogens usually do not.

CRYPTOCOCCOSIS

Disease elicited by *Cryptococcus neoformans*. The primary illness results from inhalation of the fungus in bird droppings. If the patient is debilitated, infection spreads from the lungs to the brain and rest of the body.

CUTANEOUS MYCOSIS

Fungal disease of the skin, hair, and nail. There is more tissue destruction than with a superficial mycosis.

DEMATIACEOUS

Hyphae and/or conidia in varieties of black, when observed under the microscope. In this text, drawings of dematiaceous organisms are shaded gray.

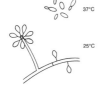

DENTICLE

Very small, hairlike stalk.

DERMATOMYCOSIS

Fungal disease affecting hair, skin, or nail.

DERMATOPHYTOSIS

Fungal disease of the hair, skin, and nail specifically caused by the genera *Epidermophyton, Microsporum,* and *Trichophyton.*

DERMATOPHYTE

Fungus infecting the dermis (hair, skin, or nail), and belonging to the genus *Epidermophyton, Microsporum* or *Trichophyton.*

DEUTEROMYCOTA

Fungal phylum in which the sexual stage does not exist or is unknown; also called Fungi Imperfecti.

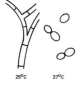

DIMORPHISM

Possessing two different appearances, or phases. In this text, the term will be limited to a mold phase at room temperature and a yeast (tissue) phase at 37°C.

DISJUNCTOR CELL

Empty cell between conidia that breaks or dissolves to release the conidia.

ECHINULATE

Having rough edges; spiny.

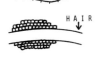

ECTOTHRIX

Infection around the outside of a hair shaft. Note that fungal invasion initially begins inside the shaft at the root, but arthroconidia develop around the outside further up. The cuticle is destroyed in this type of invasion. Ectothrix properties must be observed in specimen direct mounts, not in hairs on which fungi have been cultured in vitro.

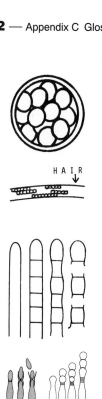

ENDOGENOUS	Originating within oneself.
ENDOSPORE	Spore produced within a spherule, as in *Coccidioides immitis*.
ENDOTHRIX	Infection with arthroconidia inside a hair shaft; the cuticle is not destroyed. Endothrix properties must be observed in specimen direct mounts, not in hairs on which fungi have been cultured in vitro.
ENTEROARTHRIC CONIDIOGENESIS	Only inner parent cell wall layers are involved in arthric daughter cell development, for example, in the arthroconidia of *Coccidioides immitis*. See ARTHRIC and THALLIC CONIDIOGENESIS.
ENTEROBLASTIC CONIDIOGENESIS	Only inner parent cell wall layers are involved in blastic daughter cell development, for example, in phialoconidia and annelloconidia. See BLASTIC CONIDIOGENESIS.
EPIDEMIOLOGY	Geographic location of a disease; also, a study to identify carriers of an infection.
ERYTHEMA	Redness.
ETIOLOGIC AGENT	Organism causing the disease.
EUKARYOTIC	Containing a true nucleus, surrounded by a nuclear membrane.
EUMYCOTIC MYCETOMA	Mycetoma caused by a true fungus. Granules of various colors may be observed, depending on the etiologic agent.
FAVIC CHANDELIERS	Blunt, branched hyphae which resemble the antlers of a buck deer. Favic chandeliers may be observed in many old cultures, but *Trichophyton schoenleinii* possesses a predominance of them.
FERMENTATION	Ability of an organism to use a compound in the absence of oxygen.
FOOT CELL	In *Aspergillus* sp. and *Apophysomyces* sp., a hyphal cell at the conidiophore base; in *Fusarium* sp., the sharply angled end of a macroconidium where it attaches to the conidiophore.
FUNGI IMPERFECTI	Those fungi whose sexual stage does not exist or has not yet been discovered. They are classified in the phylum Deuteromycota.
FUNGUS (pl. fungi)	Kingdom of organisms that contain true nuclei, are devoid of chlorophyll, and absorb all nutrients from the environment, especially decaying organic matter. Fungi may reproduce asexually and/or sexually.
FUNGUS BALL	Walled-off fungal abscess in the lungs. It may erode into surrounding blood vessels, with subsequent dis-

semination. Several genera may produce fungus balls, but the most common are *Aspergillus* and *Scedosporium*.

FUNGUSLIKE BACTERIUM

A bacterium, 1 μm in diameter, which may develop conidia and elicit a funguslike disease.

GENICULATE

Bent-knee growth; when one conidium has formed, the growing point of the hyphal strand continues in the opposite direction. The terms sympodial and geniculate usually go hand in hand.

GLABROUS TEXTURE

Colony containing no aerial hyphae. These are usually yeasts.

GRANULAR TEXTURE

Conidia in a dense profusion on top of the colony, resembling sugar granules.

GRANULE

1–2 mm-wide clump of hyphae and swollen cells in a compact mass, or funguslike bacteria radiating out from a center of necrotic debris. A cementlike matrix may be present. Granules are variously colored, depending on the etiologic agent, and they are observed in tissue from patients with mycetoma.

GRANULOMATOUS

Tumorous.

HILUM (pl. hila)

Point of attachment.

HISTOPLASMOSIS

Infection with *Histoplasma capsulatum*. Initially a subclinical respiratory infection, it becomes systemic and serious if the patient is debilitated.

HOLOARTHRIC CONIDIOGENESIS

All parent cell wall layers are involved in arthric daughter cell development, for example, the arthroconidia of *Geotrichum* sp. See ARTHRIC and THALLIC CONIDIOGENESIS.

HOLOBLASTIC CONIDIOGENESIS

All parent cell wall layers are involved in blastic daughter cell development, for example, in blastoconidia and poroconidia. See BLASTIC CONIDIOGENESIS.

HOLOTHALLIC CONIDIOGENESIS

All parent cell wall layers are involved in thallic daughter cell development, for example, in macroconidia and chlamydoconidia. See THALLIC CONIDIOGENESIS.

HYALINE

Hyphae and conidia lightly pigmented when observed under the microscope. This includes shades of blue and green.

HYALOHYPHOMYCOSIS

Infection caused by hyaline fungi and identified by the presence of light-colored hyphae in infected tissue.

HYPHA (pl. hyphae)	Long strand of cells, with or without crosswalls.

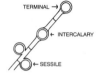

IMPERFECT FUNGI	See FUNGI IMPERFECTI.
INDURATION	Hardness.
INFLAMMATORY	Pus cell response.
INTERCALARY	Arising within the hyphal strand.
INTERMEDIATE GROWTH RATE	Forming a mature colony in 6–10 days.
IN VITRO	Outside the host, as on artificial media.
IN VIVO	Inside the host.
KERATOMYCOSIS	Opportunistic fungal infection of the cornea of the eye.
LUMPY JAW	Hard, swollen area of the jaw caused by infection with *Actinomyces*. It usually occurs after a tooth extraction.
MACROALEURIOSPORE	See MACROCONIDIUM.

MACROCONIDIUM (pl. macroconidia)	Holothallic multicelled conidium in which an entire hyphal element converts into a macroconidium. The prefix macro- should be used only when smaller microconidia are also present. Macroconidia may be thick-walled or thin-walled; smooth or rough; club-shaped, spindle-shaped, or oval; and alone or in clusters.

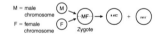

MEIOSIS	Nuclear and cytoplasmic reduction division in which a diploid zygote produces haploid daughters, each containing genetic information from both parents. This is observed in sexual reproduction.

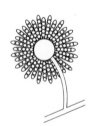

MEROSPORANGIUM	Tubelike sporangium containing sporangiospores in a row. Merosporangia are observed in *Syncephalastrum* sp.
METULA (pl. metulae)	Terminal branched conidiophore, as in *Penicillium*.
MICROALEURIOSPORE	See MICROCONIDIUM.
MICROCONIDIUM (pl. microconidia)	Holothallic single-celled (or rarely two-celled) conidium in which an entire hyphal element converts into the microconidium. The prefix micro- should be used only when larger macroconidia are also present. Microconidia are round, oval, or club-shaped, and single or in clusters.

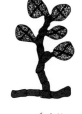

N = nonsexual chromosome (N) → (N) + (N)

MITOSIS

Nuclear and cytoplasmic division in which the two daughter cells contain the same genetic information as one parent. This occurs with multiplying, nonsexual cells, for example, skin cells in humans. In mycology, besides hyphal proliferation, mitosis is observed in asexual reproduction.

MOLD

Colony growing hyphal (as opposed to yeast) forms.

MONILIASIS

See CANDIDIASIS, CANDIDOSIS.

MURIFORM

Divided by horizontal and vertical cross septa.

MYCELIA STERILIA

No reproductive structures present, only septate hyphae. These organisms are usually of the phylum Basidiomycota; look for clamp connections. With the proper environmental conditions, e.g., different media, temperature, or atmosphere, fruiting structures should develop.

MYCELIUM (pl. mycelia)

Many hyphae intertwined to form a thick mat.

MYCETOMA

Slow-growing, subcutaneous lesion, usually on an extremity, characterized by bone deformity and oozing sinus tracts containing granules. Eumycotic mycetoma is caused by true fungi, while actinomycotic mycetoma is elicited by funguslike bacteria.

MYCOLOGY

Study of fungi.

MYCOSIS (pl. mycoses)

Disease caused by a fungus.

MYCOTIC KERATITIS

See KERATOMYCOSIS.

NECROSIS

Dead and decaying tissue.

NEUROTROPIC

Propensity to invade nervous tissue, particularly the brain.

NOCARDIOSIS

Abscess of the lungs with *Nocardia* sp. and subsequent spread to other body sites. Granules are usually not observed.

NODULAR ORGAN

Knot of twisted hyphae seen in older cultures.

ONTOGENY

Study of the maturation of an organism.

ONYCHOMYCOSIS

Fungal infection of the nail by molds or yeasts. With yeast invasion, the surrounding skin will also be affected. Other names for onychomycosis are tinea unguium, ringworm of the nail, and dermatophytosis of the nail.

OPPORTUNISTIC PATHOGEN

Not normally disease producing. When the host is debilitated, as with chronic disease, anticancer therapy, antibiotics, steroids, and so forth, the opportunists proliferate and elicit an infection.

OTOMYCOSIS

Opportunistic fungal infection of the outer ear; the inner ear is not affected.

PARACOCCIDIOIDOMYCOSIS

Infection with *Paracoccidioides brasiliensis*. The most common sites are the oral mucosa, lungs, and intestines. Lymphatic enlargement is characteristic, and with time, the disease becomes systemic.

PATHOGENIC

Producing disease.

PENICILLUS (pl. penicilli)

Conidiophores that branch in multiple layers, providing a brushlike appearance.

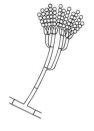

PERFECT FUNGI

Those fungi which reproduce sexually. This includes the phyla Zygomycota, Basidiomycota, and Ascomycota.

PHAEOHYPHOMYCOSIS

Formerly called chromoblastomycosis in part, cladosporiosis. Phaeohyphomycosis is a cutaneous, subcutaneous, or systemic abscess, particularly in the brain, characterized in histologic sections by dark, branched hyphae and, occasionally, spherical cells. Sclerotic bodies and granules are absent. The primary etiologic agent is *Cladosporium trichoides*.

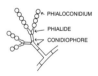

PHIALIDE

Tube-shaped or vase-shaped conidiogenous cell. The first phialoconidium is holoblastic and the rest are enteroblastic, arising from a fixed locus in the phialide. The phialide may be ringed at the top by a cup-shaped collarette.

PHIALOCONIDIUM (pl. phialoconidia)

Conidium arising from a phialide. The first develops holoblastically, but the succeeding conidia are enteroblastically derived. See drawing at PHIALIDE.

PITYRIASIS VERSICOLOR

Formerly tinea versicolor. Pityriasis versicolor is a superficial skin infection characterized by scaly patches of reddish brown, brown, and white, caused by *Malassezia furfur*.

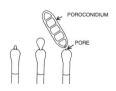

POROCONIDIUM (pl. poroconidia)

Holoblastic conidium produced through a pore in the parent cell wall.

POWDERY TEXTURE

Conidia in profusion on top of a colony, resembling flour.

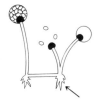

PSEUDOHYPHA

Elongated blastoconidium made by some yeast species. Cells of pseudohyphae are constricted at their points of attachment, while those of true hyphae are not.

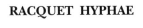

RACQUET HYPHAE

Hyphae resembling tennis racquets placed end to end, often seen in older cultures.

RAPID GROWTH RATE

Forming a mature colony within 5 days.

RHIZOID

Rootlike hypha.

RINGWORM

Common name for a fungal infection caused by *Epidermophyton, Microsporum,* or *Trichophyton.* See DERMATOPHYTOSIS.

RUGOSE TOPOGRAPHY

Furrows radiating out from the colony center.

SAN JOAQUIN VALLEY FEVER

See COCCIDIOIDOMYCOSIS.

SAPROBE

Organism able to live on decaying organic matter in the soil. Most opportunistic fungi are saprobes.

SCLEROTIC BODY

Black dot; thick-walled cell in tissue that may be divided into horizontal and/or vertical cross septa. Sclerotic bodies are observed in chromoblastomycosis.

SEPTATE

Containing cross-walls in hyphae, conidia, or spores.

SEPTUM (pl. septa)

Cross-wall in a hypha, spore, or conidium; it usually contains a septal pore, allowing some movement of the cellular contents from one cell to another.

SEROLOGY

Study of antigen and antibody reactions.

SEROMYCOLOGY

Study of fungal antigens and antibodies.

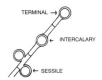

SESSILE

Arising on the sides of a hypha.

SEXUAL REPRODUCTION

Fusion of two compatible haploid nuclei to form a zygote.

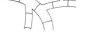

SHIELD CELL

Conidiogenous cell that gives rise to two branches of reproductive structures. Scars at the branch point of attachment give the conidiogenous cell a shield appearance. These cells are observed in *Cladosporium* sp.

SINUS TRACT

In mycetoma and actinomycosis, a tunnel eroded from the infected site to a drainage area, for example, from the lungs to the skin.

SLOW GROWTH RATE

Forming a mature colony in 11–21 days.

SOUTH AMERICAN BLASTOMYCOSIS

See PARACOCCIDIOIDOMYCOSIS.

SPHERULE

Thick-walled spherical structure produced in tissue or under special in vitro conditions by *Coccidioides immitis.* When young, the spherules are empty; with age, they become filled with endospores.

SPINDLE-SHAPED

Enlarged in the middle and tapered at the ends, resembling a spindle of yarn on a spinning wheel.

SPIRAL HYPHA

Hypha curved in a spiral, either flat or like a corkscrew.

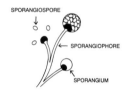

SPORANGIOPHORE

Asexual stalk that supports a sporangium. It may be branched or unbranched.

SPORANGIOSPORE

Asexual spore formed by cleavage of the sporangium contents. Sporangiospores are produced by the phylum Zygomycota. See drawing at SPORANGIOPHORE.

SPORANGIUM (pl. sporangia)

Asexual saclike structure at the tip of a sporangiophore, with developing sporangiospores inside. See drawing at SPORANGIOPHORE.

SPORODCHIUM

Hyphal mat densely covered with short conidiophores and conidia.

SPOROTRICHOSIS

Subcutaneous, hard, black, ulcerating lesions, usually on the extremities, caused by *Sporothrix schenckii.* Granules are not observed.

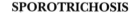
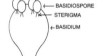

STERIGMA (pl. sterigmata)

This term is now reserved for the structure that supports a basidiospore on top of a basidium. Regarding *Aspergillus* and *Penicillium,* sterigmata have been replaced by the term phialides.

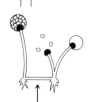

STOLON

Hyphal runner connecting groups of sporangiophores, similar to the runner that connects raspberry bushes.

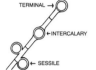

SUBCUTANEOUS MYCOSIS	Fungal disease of the skin, muscle, and connective tissue immediately beneath the skin.
SUPERFICIAL MYCOSIS	Fungal disease of the outermost layers of skin and hair, with little or no pathology evidenced.
SYMPODIAL	First developing a conidium on one side, then further up on the other side, in a repetitive fashion. The hyphal stalk may be straight or in a bent-knee type of arrangement.
SYSTEMIC MYCOSIS	Fungal disease of the deep tissues and organs of the body. In disseminated forms of these infections, subcutaneous and cutaneous areas may also be invaded.
TAXONOMY	Classification of organisms by kingdoms, divisions, subdivisions, classes, orders, families, genera, and species.
TELEOMORPH	Sexual name.
TERMINAL	At the (hyphal) tip.
TEXTURE	Term to describe the height of aerial hyphae on a colony.
THALLIC CONIDIOGENESIS	A septum forms near the end of a parent, and the growing point ahead of it becomes the daughter conidium. The daughter develops *after* it is separated, although still attached to the parent. Thallic development may be holothallic or arthric.
THROMBOSIS	Blood clot with subsequent necrosis of surrounding tissue due to lack of oxygen.
THRUSH	Candidiasis of the oral cavity, usually observed in infants of mothers with vaginal candidiasis, and in elderly debilitated patients.
TINEA	Dermatophytosis.
TINEA BARBAE	Dermatophytosis of the beard; barber's itch.
TINEA CAPITIS	Dermatophytosis of the scalp.
TINEA CORPORIS	Dermatophytosis of the body.
TINEA CRURIS	Dermatophytosis of the groin; jock itch.
TINEA NIGRA	Superficial skin infection, usually on the palms of the hands, characterized by nonscaly brown to black patches, and caused by *Exophiala werneckii.*
TINEA PEDIS	Dermatophytosis of the foot; athlete's foot.
TINEA UNGUIUM	Dermatophytosis of the nail; onychomycosis.
TINEA VERSICOLOR	See PITYRIASIS VERSICOLOR.
TOPOGRAPHY	Design of hills and valleys observed on fungal colonies.
TRUNCATE	Having a squared-off appearance.

UMBONATE

AERIAL ← CONIDIA
← SURFACE OF AGAR
(CROSS SECTION)
VEGETATIVE

UMBONATE TOPOGRAPHY

Buttonlike central elevation on a fungal colony, often accompanied by rugose furrows.

VEGETATIVE

Food-absorbing portion of the hyphae, which grow into the agar like roots. Vegetative hyphae may best be seen on the colony's reverse side.

VELVETY TEXTURE

Colonial aerial hyphae arising close and parallel to each other, approximately ¼ inch high, and resembling the fabric velvet.

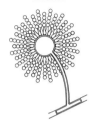

VERRUCOSE

VERRUCOSE TOPOGRAPHY

Deeply wrinkled, convoluted colony surface.

VESICLE

Swollen hypha. It may be the tip of a conidiophore as in *Aspergillus* sp., or the end of a sporangiophore as in *Syncephalastrum* sp.

WHITE PIEDRA

Light-brown soft nodules around beard and mustache hairs, caused by *Trichosporon beigelii*.

WHORL

Several conidia or conidiophores forming around a common axis.

WOOLLY TEXTURE

Colonial aerial hyphae with a slightly matted appearance, approximately ½ inch high, resembling wool.

YEAST

Single round to oval cell that usually buds to form daughter cells.

ZYGOMYCETOUS

Pertaining to the taxonomic phylum Zygomycota.

ZYGOMYCOSIS

Opportunistic fungal infection caused by genera of the phylum Zygomycota. Usually the acute form is elicited in which the initial eye or nasal sinus infection erodes into surrounding tissues, with rapid spread and death.

ZYGOMYCOTA

Fungal phylum exhibiting hyphae 6–10 μm wide which are aseptate, except at damaged areas or reproductive structures. Sporangiospores are the typical asexual stage, while zygospores are formed sexually.

IMMATURE

MATURE ZYGOSPORANGIUM

ZYGOPHORE

Arm of a hypha that extends toward another compatible arm to produce a zygospore. These are seen in the phylum Zygomycota.

ZYGOSPORANGIUM

Thick outer layer covering a zygospore seen in the Zygomycota. See drawing at ZYGOPHORE.

ZYGOSPORE

Sexual spore formed by meeting and fusion of two compatible hyphal arms, each containing a nucleus. The resulting zygote becomes a zygospore and is surrounded by a protective zygosporangium. These structures are observed in the phylum Zygomycota. See drawing at ZYGOPHORE.

APPENDIX

List of Manufacturers

ABBOTT LABORATORIES
One Abbott Park Road
Abbott Park, IL 60064-3500
(708)937-3280

BAXTER DIAGNOSTICS INC.
See DADE INTERNATIONAL

BBL
See BECTON DICKINSON AND
COMPANY

BECTON DICKINSON AND COMPANY
1 Becton Drive
Franklin Lakes, NJ 07417-1880
(201)847-6670

BECTON DICKINSON DIAGNOSTIC
INSTRUMENT SYSTEMS
7 Loveton Circle
Sparks, MD 21152
(410)316-4000
(800)638-8656

BECTON DICKINSON
IMMUNODIAGNOSTICS
Mountainview Avenue
Orangeburg, NY 10962
(914)359-2700
(800)431-1237

BECTON DICKINSON
MICROBIOLOGY SYSTEMS
250 Schilling Circle, P.O. Box 243
Cockeysville, MD 21030
(410)584-8977
Fax (410)584-2806

BIOMÉRIEUX VITEK, INC.
595 Anglum Drive
Hazelwood, MO 63042
(314)731-8504
(800)638-4835
Fax (314)731-8700

BIOWHITTAKER, INC.
8830 Biggs Ford Road (A08)
Walkersville, MD 21793-0127
(301)898-7025

CARR-SCARBOROUGH
MICROBIOLOGICALS, INC.
5342 Panola Industrial Boulevard
Decatur, GA 30035
(404)987-9300

CLINICAL STANDARDS
LABORATORIES, INC.
2011 E. University Drive
Rancho Dominguez, CA 90220-6445
(310)537-6800

DADE INTERNATIONAL INC.
1717 Deerfield Road
Deerfield, IL 60015
(708)267-5423
Fax (708)267-5433

DADE MICROSCAN
1584 Enterprise Avenue
West Sacramento, CA 95691
(916)372-1900
Fax (916)372-2081

DIFCO LABORATORIES
P.O. Box 331058
Detroit, MI 48232-7058
(313)462-8500

GEN-PROBE INCORPORATED
9880 Campus Point Drive
San Diego, CA 92121
(619)546-7978

IMMUNO-MYCOLOGICS, INC.
P.O. Box 1151
Norman, OK 73070
(405)288-2383

INNOVATIVE DIAGNOSTIC SYSTEMS, INC.
2797 Peterson Place
Norcross, GA 30071
(800)225-5443

INTERNATIONAL BIOLOGICAL LABORATORIES
See WAMPOLE LABORATORIES

MARION SCIENTIFIC
See BECTON DICKINSON AND COMPANY

MEDICAL WIRE & EQUIPMENT CO. (USA)
7 The Boardwalk
Sparta, NJ 07871
(800)321-3244

MERIDIAN DIAGNOSTICS, INC.
3471 River Hills Drive
Cincinnati, OH 45244
(513)271-3700

MUREX DIAGNOSTICS, INC.
3075 Northwoods Circle
Norcross, GA 30071
(404)662-0660
(800)448-5661
Fax (404)449-4018

ORGANON TEKNIKA
100 Akzo Avenue
Durham, NC 27712
(919)620-2315

PML MICROBIOLOGICALS
9595 SW Tualatin Sherwood Road
P.O. Box 459
Tualatin, OR 97062-0459
(503)692-1030

RAMCO LABORATORIES, INC.
4507 Mt. Vernon
Houston, TX 77006
(713)526-9677

REMEL
12076 Santa Fe Drive
Lenexa, KS 66215
(800)255-6730

SANOFI DIAGNOSTIC PASTEUR
1000 Lake Hazeltine Drive
Chaska, MN 55318-1084
(612)368-1124

SMITHKLINE DIAGNOSTICS, INC.
225 Baypoint Parkway
San Jose, CA 95134
(408)425-2660
(800)877-6242
Fax (408)435-7980

TRINITY LABORATORIES
7517 Precision Drive, Ste. 107
Raleigh, NC 27613
(919)598-5000

WAMPOLE LABORATORIES
Half Acre Road
P.O. Box 1001
Cranbury, NJ 08512
(609)655-6157
(800)257-9525

COLOR PLATES

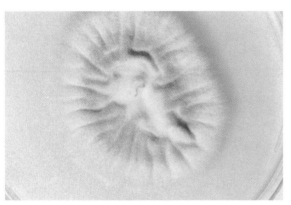

1. Colony front, *Microsporum cookei,* Sabouraud dextrose agar (SDA), 7 days, 25°C.

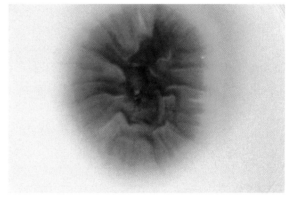

2. Colony reverse, *Microsporum cookei,* SDA, 7 days, 25°C.

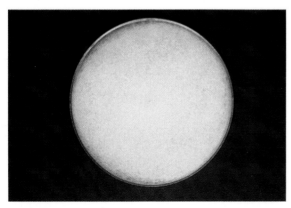

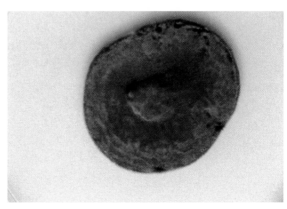

3. Cottony texture, *Rhizopus* sp., SDA, 3 days, 25°C.

4. Velvety texture, *Fonsecaea pedrosoi,* SDA, 16 days, 25°C.

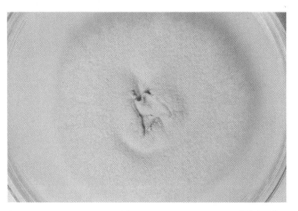

5. Powdery texture, *Microsporum gypseum*, SDA, 7 days, 25°C.

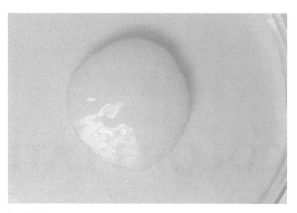

6. Glabrous texture, *Cryptococcus neoformans*, SDA, 17 days, 25°C.

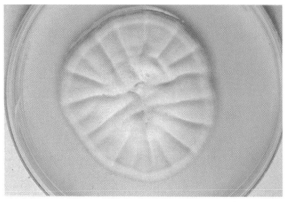

7. Rugose topography, *Epidermophyton floccosum*, SDA, 14 days, 25°C.

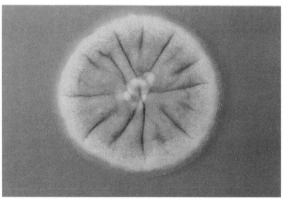

8. Umbonate and rugose topography, *Aspergillus fumigatus*, SDA, 5 days, 25°C.

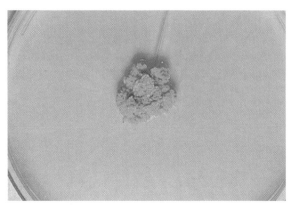

9. Verrucose topography, *Nocardia asteroides*, SDA, 18 days, 25°C.

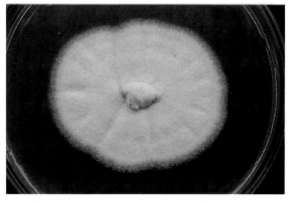

10. Module 1 final exam photograph, colony front.

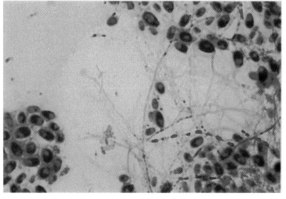

11. Module 1 final exam photograph, colony reverse.

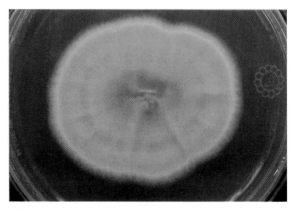

12. Modified Kinyoun carbolfuchsin acid-fast stain, *Nocardia* sp., ×1000.

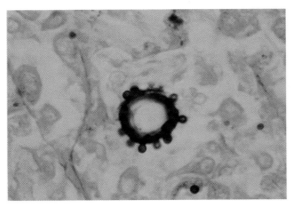

13. Gomori methenamine silver stain, *Paracoccidioides brasiliensis*, ×1000.

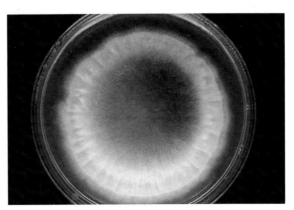

14. *Absidia* sp., SDA, 4 days, 25°C.

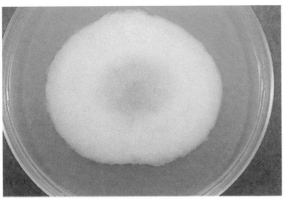

15. *Mucor* sp., SDA, 10 days, 25°C.

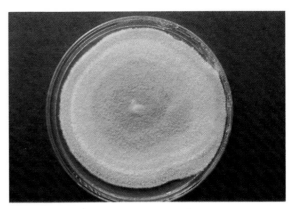

16. *Alternaria* sp., SDA, 9 days, 25°C.

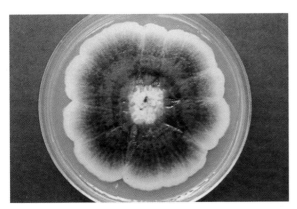

17. *Aureobasidium* sp., SDA, 14 days, 25°C.

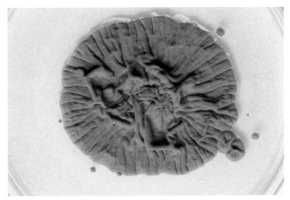

18. *Cladosporium* sp., SDA, 10 days, 25°C.

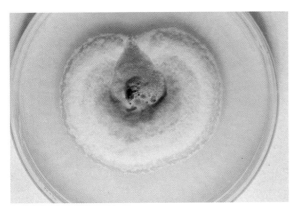

19. *Curvularia* sp., SDA, 6 days, 25°C.

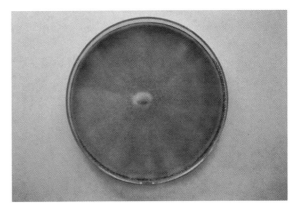

20. *Drechslera* sp., SDA, 14 days, 25°C.

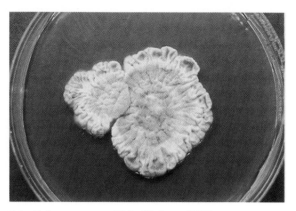

21. *Epicoccum* sp., SDA, 13 days, 25°C.

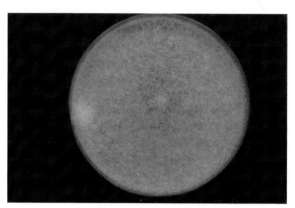

22. *Nigrospora* sp., SDA, 6 days, 25°C.

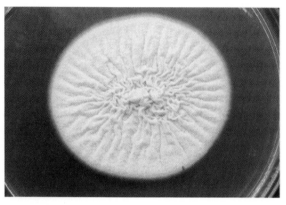

23. *Acremonium* sp., SDA, 13 days, 25°C.

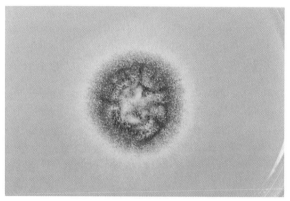

24. *Aspergillus niger*, SDA, 3 days, 25°C.

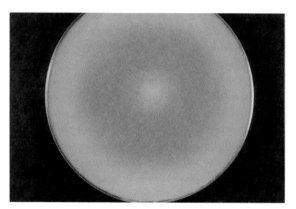

25. *Syncephalastrum* sp., SDA, 5 days, 25°C.

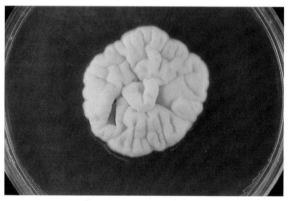

26. *Chrysosporium* sp., SDA, 8 days, 25°C.

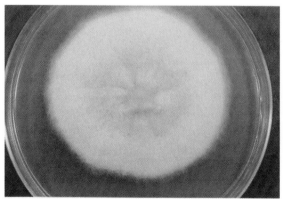

27. *Fusarium* sp., SDA, 9 days, 25°C.

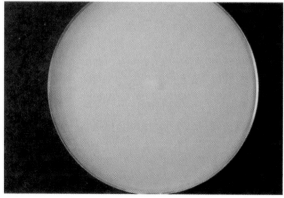

28. *Gliocladium* sp., SDA, 5 days, 25°C.

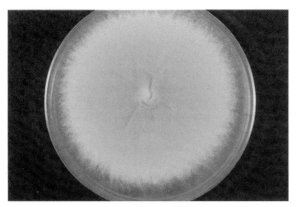

29. *Paecilomyces* sp., SDA, 5 days, 25°C.

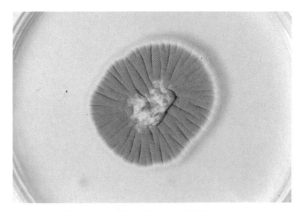

30. *Penicillium* sp., SDA, 6 days, 25°C.

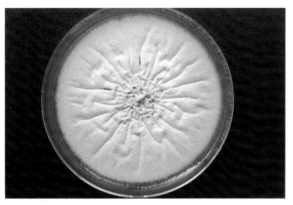

31. *Scopulariopsis,* sp., SDA, 14 days, 25°C.

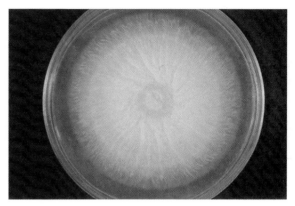

32. *Sepedonium* sp., SDA, 5 days, 25°C.

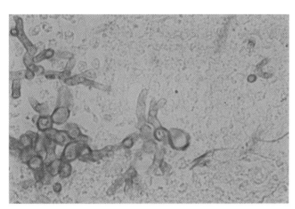

33. Aspergillosis of lung, Gridley fungus stain, ×450.

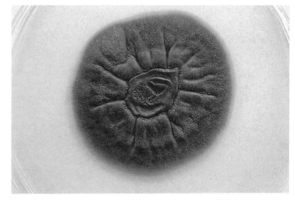

34. *Exophiala werneckii*, SDA, 39 days, 25°C.

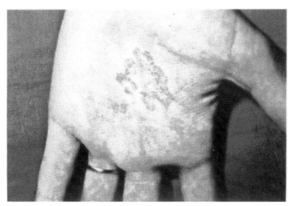

35. Tinea nigra. (From Beneke: Human Mycoses. Upjohn, 1979, with permission.)

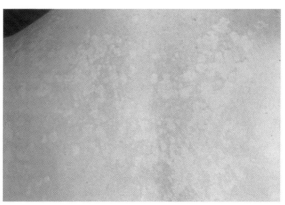

36. Pityriasis versicolor. (From Beneke: Human Mycoses. Upjohn, 1979, with permission.)

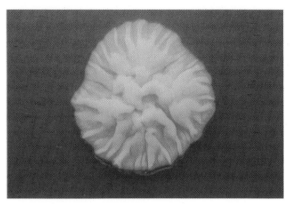

37. *Trichosporon beigelii*, SDA, 10 days, 25°C.

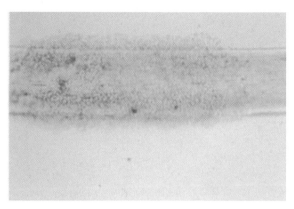

38. White piedra, hair, ×200 (Center for Disease Control).

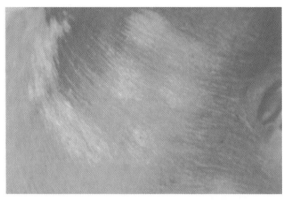

39. Fluorescing hair. (From Dolan et al: Atlas of Clinical Mycology. ASCP, 1976, with permission.)

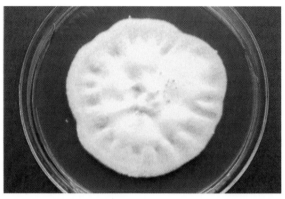

40. *Microsporum audouinii*, SDA, 39 days, 25°C.

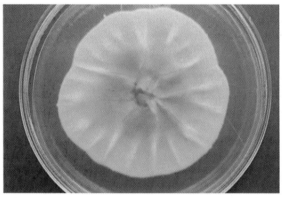

41. Colony reverse, *Microsporum audouinii*, SDA, 39 days, 25°C.

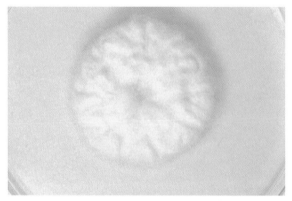

42. *Microsporum canis*, SDA, 7 days, 25°C.

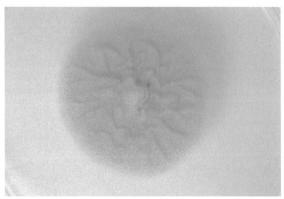

43. Colony reverse, *Microsporum canis*, SDA, 7 days, 25°C.

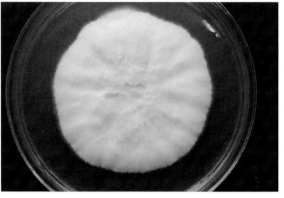

44. Fluffy strain, *Trichophyton mentagrophytes*, SDA, 20 days, 25°C.

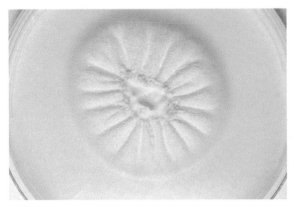

45. Granular strain, *Trichophyton mentagrophytes*, SDA, 10 days, 25°C.

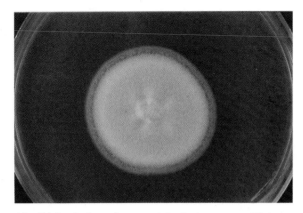

46. *Trichophyton rubrum*, potato dextrose agar, 16 days, 25°C.

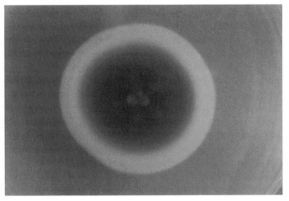

47. Colony reverse, *Trichophyton rubrum*, potato dextrose agar, 16 days, 25°C.

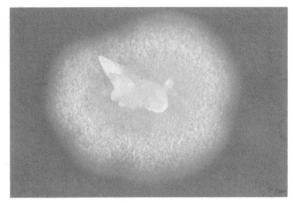

48. *Trichophyton verrucosum*, SDA, 28 days, 37°C.

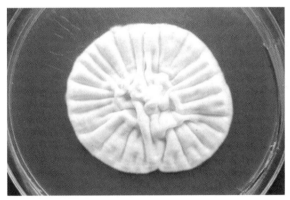

49. *Trichophyton schoenleinii*, SDA, 39 days, 25°C.

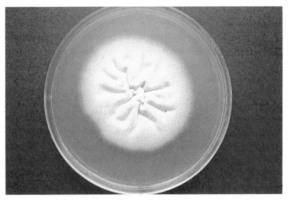

50. *Trichophyton tonsurans*, SDA, 28 days, 25°C.

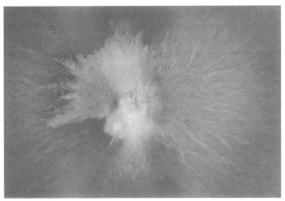

51. *Trichophyton violaceum*, SDA, 28 days, 25°C.

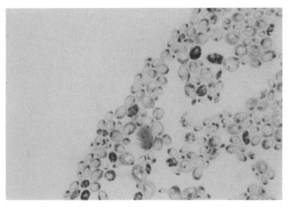

52. Ascus containing two ascospores, *Saccharomyces cerevisiae*, modified Kinyoun acid-fast stain, ×1000.

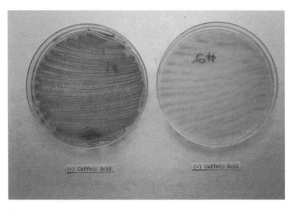

53. Caffeic acid agar: (+) test, *Cryptococcus neoformans;* (−) test, *Candida albicans.*

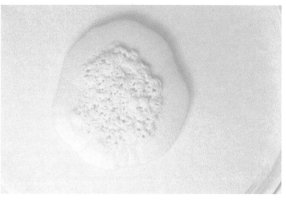

54. *Candida albicans,* SDA, 17 days, 25°C.

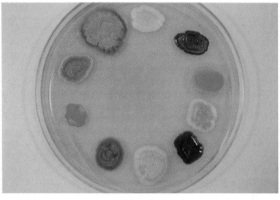

55. Candida BCG agar, 3 days, 25°C (clockwise starting at top): *Candida albicans, Candida (Torulopsis) glabrata, Candida krusei, Candida parapsilosis, Candida pseudotropicalis, Candida tropicalis, Cryptococcus neoformans, Prototheca, Saccharomyces cerevisiae, Trichosporon beigelii.*

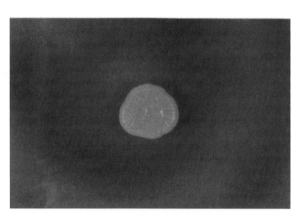

56. Module 5 final exam photograph.

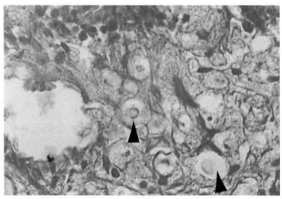

57. Cryptococcosis of lung, hematoxylin and eosin stain, ×450. Arrows indicate the capsule surrounding the organism.

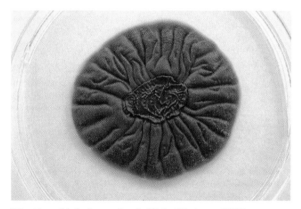

58. *Exophiala jeanselmei,* SDA, 39 days, 25°C.

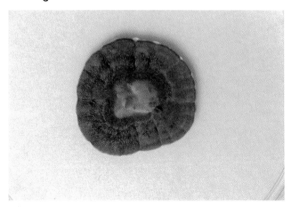

59. *Phialophora verrucosa,* SDA, 20 days, 25°C.

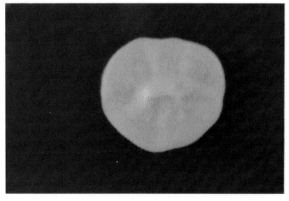

60. *Scedosporium apiospermum,* SDA, 8 days, 25°C.

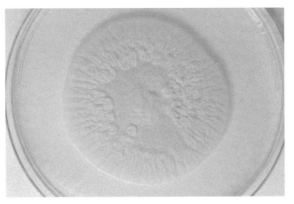

61. *Sporothrix schenckii*, SDA, 23 days, 25°C.

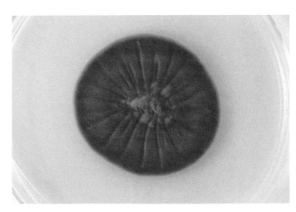

62. *Sporothrix schenckii*, potato dextrose agar, 19 days, 25°C.

63. *Sporothrix schenckii*, brain heart infusion agar with blood, 14 days, 37°C.

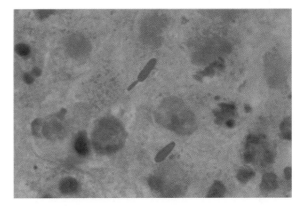

64. *Sporothrix schenckii* yeasts in hand aspirate, periodic acid-Schiff stain, ×1000.

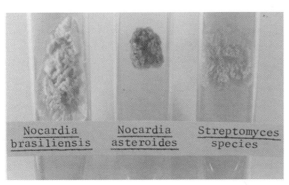

65. *Nocardia brasiliensis, Nocardia asteroides,* and *Streptomyces* sp., SDA, 21 days, 25°C.

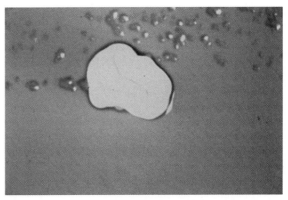

66. Molar tooth colony, *Actinomyces.* (From Dolan et al: Atlas of Clinical Mycology. ASCP, 1976, with permission.)

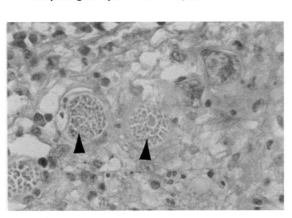

67. *Coccidioides immitis* spherules, hematoxylin and eosin stain, ×450. Arrows indicate spherules.

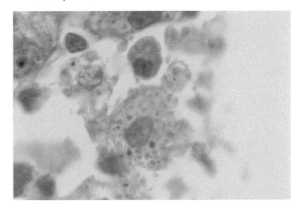

68. Yeasts of *Histoplasma capsulatum* inside spleen macrophage (center of photo), hematoxylin and eosin stain, ×1000.

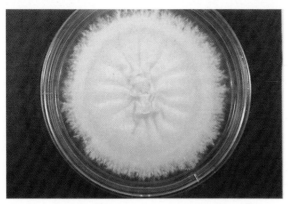

69. *Blastomyces dermatitidis*, SDA, 42 days, 25°C.

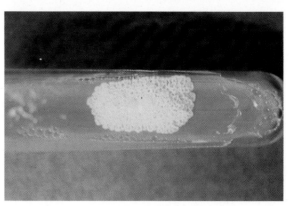

70. *Blastomyces dermatitidis*, brain heart infusion agar with blood, 14 days, 37°C.

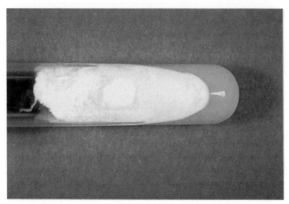

71. *Coccidioides immitis*, SDA, 28 days, 25°C.

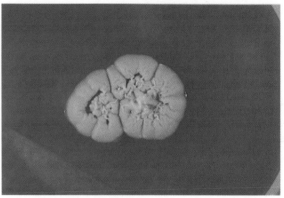

72. *Histoplasma capsulatum*, brain heart infusion agar with blood, 21 days, 25°C.

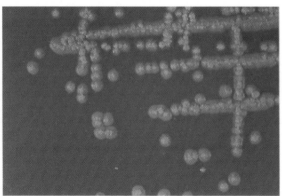

73. *Histoplasma capsulatum*, brain heart infusion agar with blood, 14 days, 37°C.

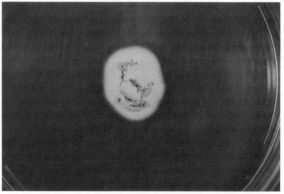

74. *Paracoccidioides brasiliensis*, SDA, 42 days, 25°C.

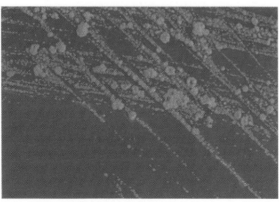

75. *Paracoccidioides brasiliensis*, brain heart infusion agar with blood, 14 days, 37°C.

Index